Allergy for the Otolaryngologist

Editors

MURUGAPPAN RAMANATHAN Jr
JAMES W. MIMS

OTOLARYNGOLOGIC CLINICS OF NORTH AMERICA

www.oto.theclinics.com

Consulting Editor
SUJANA S. CHANDRASEKHAR

December 2017 • Volume 50 • Number 6

ELSEVIER

1600 John F. Kennedy Boulevard • Suite 1800 • Philadelphia, Pennsylvania, 19103-2899

http://www.oto.theclinics.com

OTOLARYNGOLOGIC CLINICS OF NORTH AMERICA Volume 50, Number 6
December 2017 ISSN 0030-6665, ISBN-13: 978-0-323-58314-5

Editor: Jessica McCool
Developmental Editor: Alison Swety

Otolaryngologic Clinics of North America (ISSN 0030-6665) is published bimonthly by Elsevier, Inc., 360 Park Avenue South, New York, NY 10010-1710. Months of issue are February, April, June, August, October, and December. Business and Editorial Offices: 1600 John F. Kennedy Blvd., Suite 1800, Philadelphia, PA 19103-2899. Customer Service Office: 6277 Sea Harbor Drive, Orlando, FL 32887-4800. Periodicals postage paid at New York, NY and additional mailing offices. Subscription prices are $381.00 per year (US individuals), $803.00 per year (US institutions), $100.00 per year (US student/resident), $500.00 per year (Canadian individuals), $1017.00 per year (Canadian institutions), $556.00 per year (international individuals), $1017.00 per year (international institutions), $270.00 per year (international & Canadian student/resident). Foreign air speed delivery is included in all *Clinics'* subscription prices. All prices are subject to change without notice. **POSTMASTER:** Send address changes to *Otolaryngologic Clinics of North America*, Elsevier Health Sciences Division, Subscription Customer Service, 3251 Riverport Lane, Maryland Heights, MO 63043. **Telephone: 1-800-654-2452 (U.S. and Canada); 314-447-8871 (outside U.S. and Canada). Fax: 314-447-8029. E-mail: journalscustomerservice-usa@elsevier.com (for print support); journalsonlinesupport-usa@elsevier.com (for online support).**

Reprints. For copies of 100 or more of articles in this publication, please contact the Commercial Reprints Department, Elsevier Inc., 360 Park Avenue South, New York, NY 10010-1710. Tel.: 212-633-3874; Fax: 212-633-3820; E-mail: reprints@elsevier.com.

Otolaryngologic Clinics of North America is also published in Spanish by McGraw-Hill Interamericana Editores S.A., P.O. Box 5-237, 06500 Mexico D.F., Mexico.

Otolaryngologic Clinics of North America is covered in *MEDLINE/PubMed (Index Medicus), Current Contents/Clinical Medicine, Excerpta Medica, BIOSIS, Science Citation Index,* and *ISI/BIOMED.*

TO ENROLL

To enroll in the *Otolaryngologic Clinics of North America* Continuing Medical Education program, call customer service at 1-800-654-2452 or sign up online at http://www.theclinics.com/home/cme. The CME program is available to subscribers for an additional annual fee of USD 260.

METHOD OF PARTICIPATION

In order to claim credit, participants must complete the following:

1. Complete enrolment as indicated above.
2. Read the activity.
3. Complete the CME Test and Evaluation. Participants must achieve a score of 70% on the test. All CME Tests and Evaluations must be completed online.

CME INQUIRIES/SPECIAL NEEDS

For all CME inquiries or special needs, please contact elsevierCME@elsevier.com.

Contributors

CONSULTING EDITOR

SUJANA S. CHANDRASEKHAR, MD
Director, New York Otology; Clinical Professor of Otolaryngology-HNS, Hofstra-Northwell School of Medicine, Hempstead, New York; Clinical Associate Professor of Otolaryngology-HNS, Mount Sinai School of Medicine, New York, New York

EDITORS

MURUGAPPAN RAMANATHAN Jr, MD, FACS
Director, National Capitol Region, Associate Professor, Rhinology and Endoscopic Skull Base Surgery, Departments of Otolaryngology, Head and Neck Surgery and Neurosurgery, The Johns Hopkins University School of Medicine, Bethesda, Maryland

JAMES W. MIMS, MD
Associate Professor, Department of Otolaryngology, Wake Forest Baptist Health, Winston-Salem, North Carolina

AUTHORS

CHRISTOPHER D. BROOK, MD
Department of Otolaryngology–Head and Neck Surgery, Boston University Medical Campus, Boston, Massachusetts

CECELIA DAMASK, DO, FAAOA
Private Practice, Florida Hospital Altamonte, Springs, Florida; Assistant Professor, Department of Otolaryngology, College of Medicine, University of Central Florida, Lake Mary ENT and Allergy, Lake Mary, Florida

THOMAS S. EDWARDS, MD
Resident Physician, Department of Otolaryngology–Head and Neck Surgery, Emory Sinus, Nasal & Allergy Center, Emory University, Atlanta, Georgia

CHRISTINE B. FRANZESE, MD, FAAOA
Department of Otolaryngology–Head and Neck Surgery, Professor, Director of Allergy, University of Missouri Medical Center-Columbia, Columbia, Missouri

SAIED GHADERSOHI, MD
Department of Otolaryngology–Head and Neck Surgery, Northwestern University Feinberg School of Medicine, Chicago, Illinois

ASHLEIGH A. HALDERMAN, MD
Assistant Professor, Department of Otolaryngology–Head and Neck Surgery, The University of Texas Southwestern Medical Center, Dallas, Texas

JOHN H. KROUSE, MD, PhD, MBA
Vice President for Medical Affairs, Dean, The University of Texas Rio Grande Valley School of Medicine, Edinburg, Texas

STELLA E. LEE, MD
Assistant Professor, Department of Otolaryngology–Head and Neck Surgery, University of Pittsburgh Medical Center, Mercy Hospital, Pittsburgh, Pennsylvania

SANDRA Y. LIN, MD
Department of Otolaryngology–Head and Neck Surgery, The Johns Hopkins University School of Medicine, Baltimore, Maryland

NYALL R. LONDON Jr, MD, PhD
Department of Otolaryngology–Head and Neck Surgery, The Johns Hopkins University School of Medicine, Baltimore, Maryland

AMBER U. LUONG, MD, PhD
Associate Professor and Director of Research, Department of Otorhinolaryngology–Head and Neck Surgery, McGovern Medical School, The University of Texas Health Science Center at Houston, Houston, Texas

MICHAEL J. MARINO, MD
Assistant Professor, Department of Otolaryngology–Head and Neck Surgery, Mayo Clinic, Phoenix, Arizona

JAMES W. MIMS, MD
Department of Otolaryngology, Wake Forest Baptist Health, Associate Professor, Department of Otolaryngology, Wake Forest School of Medicine, Winston-Salem, North Carolina

MICHAEL P. PLATT, MD, MSc
Associate Professor, Residency Program Director, Department of Otolaryngology–Head and Neck Surgery, Boston University School of Medicine, Boston, Massachusetts

MURUGAPPAN RAMANATHAN Jr, MD, FACS
Medical Director, Otolaryngology Head and Neck Surgery-National Capitol Region, Section Chief, Otolaryngology-Suburban Hospital/Johns Hopkins Medicine, Assistant Professor, Rhinology and Endoscopic Skull Base Surgery, The Johns Hopkins University School of Medicine, Baltimore, Maryland; National Capitol Region Practice, Johns Hopkins Health Care & Surgery Center/Suburban Outpatient Medical Center, Bethesda, Maryland

CHRISTOPHER R. ROXBURY, MD
Department of Otolaryngology–Head and Neck Surgery, The Johns Hopkins University School of Medicine, Baltimore, Maryland

JULIE P. SHTRAKS, MD
Department of Otolaryngology–Head and Neck Surgery, Lewis Katz School of Medicine, Temple University, Philadelphia, Pennsylvania

BRUCE K. TAN, MD, MS
Department of Otolaryngology–Head and Neck Surgery, Northwestern University Feinberg School of Medicine, Chicago, Illinois

ELINA TOSKALA, MD, PhD, MBA
Department of Otolaryngology–Head and Neck Surgery, Lewis Katz School of Medicine, Temple University, Philadelphia, Pennsylvania

LAURA J. TULLY, MD
Assistant Professor, Department of Otolaryngology–Head and Neck Surgery, The University of Texas Southwestern Medical Center, Dallas, Texas

SARAH K. WISE, MD, MSCR, FAAOA
Associate Professor, Department of Otolaryngology–Head and Neck Surgery, Emory Sinus, Nasal & Allergy Center, Emory University, Atlanta, Georgia

JACQUELINE A. WULU, MD
Department of Otolaryngology–Head and Neck Surgery, Boston University School of Medicine, Boston, Massachusetts

BETTY YANG, MD
Department of Otolaryngology–Head and Neck Surgery, Boston University Medical Campus, Boston, Massachusetts

Contents

> Recent advances in the diagnosis and management of allergic disease also lead to new clinical decisions for providers. Advances in component (or molecular) diagnostic testing for allergy continue to build in the literature, but diagnosing inhalant allergy remains largely unchanged clinically. Prevention of allergy has been demonstrated by preventing peanut allergy in high-risk infants by intentional oral exposure to promote tolerance. Immunotherapy options have increased, with literature supporting sublingual drops, sublingual tablets, and subcutaneous immunotherapy. Expanded options create clinical questions, such as the role of monotherapy in polysensitized patients. This article explores recent advances and their clinical implications.

> The sinonasal epithelial barrier is comprised of tight and adherens junction proteins. Disruption of epithelial barrier function has been hypothesized to contribute to allergic disease, such as allergic rhinitis, through increased passage of antigens and exposure of underlying tissue to these stimuli. Several mechanisms of sinonasal epithelial barrier disruption include antigen proteolytic activity, inflammatory cytokine-mediated tight junction breakdown, or exacerbation from environmental stimuli. Mechanisms of sinonasal epithelial barrier stabilization include corticosteroids and nuclear erythroid 2-related factor 2 cytoprotective pathway activation. Additional studies will aid in determining the contribution of epithelial barrier function in allergic rhinitis pathophysiology and treatment.

> The upper and lower airways are linked epidemiologically and pathophysiologically. The upper and lower airways are considered a single, functional unit characterized by shared immunologic mechanisms, often referred to as the unified airway. Upper and lower airway inflammatory disease frequently coexist in the same patient. Allergic rhinitis and rhinosinusitis are associated with asthma. Treatment of both diseases impacts

asthma outcomes. The otolaryngologist may be the first physician to suspect and diagnose asthma in patients with upper airway complaints. A thorough understanding of the relationship among allergic rhinitis, rhinosinusitis, and asthma will facilitate early identification of asthma and improve patient outcomes.

Asthma is a chronic inflammatory disease that will frequently be encountered by otolaryngologists as they manage their patients with upper respiratory diseases. Symptoms such as cough should alert otolaryngologists to consider more broadly the potential role of asthma in the differential diagnosis. It is critical for otolaryngologists to appreciate that patients with allergic rhinitis and chronic rhinosinusitis will often have asthma, and that many of them may not be diagnosed at the time of presentation. Appropriate diagnosis of the patient with asthma, as well as effective treatment for its symptoms, will improve patient function and enhance quality of life.

The role of allergy in chronic rhinosinusitis (CRS) has long been debated and remains controversial. The 2 diseases frequently co-occur; however, direct causality has never been proved. The literature is largely mixed as to the manner and degree by which allergy contributes to CRS and this is in large part due to heterogeneity in the definitions of allergy and of CRS. In this article, the potential role of allergy in the disease processes of CRS without polyps, CRS with polyps, and allergic fungal rhinosinusitis is discussed.

Allergy is commonly associated with conditions such as rhinitis, sinusitis, and asthma, but the relationship between allergy and otologic diseases is less clear. This article examines the evidence for a relationship between allergic disease and several common otologic conditions, including otitis media with effusion, eosinophilic otitis media, and Ménière's disease.

Allergy testing is commonly used when symptoms of allergic rhinitis are refractory to symptoms and there is potential for treatment with institution of avoidance measures or immunotherapy. Once the decision for testing has been made, the method of testing by either in vivo skin testing by prick/puncture or intradermal testing, or in vitro testing of serum-specific IgE is dictated by factors in the clinical history and an informed decision by the patient. Because there is no perfect testing method, understanding the benefits and limitations of each method is important in selecting the best testing option for each patient.

symptoms of allergy. Allergen immunotherapy treatment strategy for the polysensitized patient in Europe is to treat the single or 2 most clinically relevant allergen(s), whereas patients in the United States are usually treated for all potential clinically relevant allergens.

Food allergy has been increasing in prevalence for the past few decades, and numerous studies have evaluated ways of improving the allergy practitioner's ability to accurately diagnose patients who are truly food allergic, rather than sensitive but able to tolerate food. Once diagnosed, the current standard treatment is food elimination and avoidance, but other potential treatment options, like oral immunotherapy, sublingual immunotherapy, and epicutaneous immunotherapy, are becoming promising alternatives. Due to health care costs and potential for life-threatening adverse reactions, much attention has been given to the prevention of food allergies, resulting a shift in recent guideline recommendations.

Anaphylaxis is a severe systemic reaction that can be managed appropriately with expedient diagnosis and treatment. Intramuscular epinephrine continues to be the mainstay of treatment of anaphylaxis; however, it is still underused in the community and in the medical setting. Further education and counseling of patients and health care providers is required to prevent and manage anaphylaxis successfully. In-office management of anaphylaxis includes training of staff, preparedness with the necessary supplies and medication, and an effective action plan.

There are several advances in diagnosis and management for the otolaryngologist treating allergy. These include new technologies and the refinement of current techniques, and reflect overall trends in health care toward personalized medicine. Local immunoglobulin, urinary leukotriene E4, lipidomics, microRNA within extracellular vesicles, and optical rhinometry all offer to improve the diagnostic accuracy of allergy and related nonallergic conditions. New delivery systems for intranasal steroids and antihistamines, recombinant allergens, advances in allergen immunotherapy delivery, and biologics will improve current management options. These developments will aid the otolaryngologist in diagnosing and treating allergy and related diseases.

OTOLARYNGOLOGIC CLINICS
OF NORTH AMERICA

RELATED INTEREST

Immunology and Allergy Clinics of North America
February 2018 (Vol. 38, Issue 1)
Food Allergy
J. Andrew Bird, *Editor*
Available at: http://www.immunology.theclinics.com/

THE CLINICS ARE AVAILABLE ONLINE!
Access your subscription at:
www.theclinics.com

Foreword

Allergy as Part of the Unified Otolaryngologic Practice

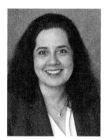

Sujana S. Chandrasekhar, MD
Consulting Editor

The management of allergic disorders is an integral part of the specialty of otolaryngology–head and neck surgery. Its importance in the comprehensive management of the ENT patient has become more and more apparent over time. In 1985, 58% of Otolaryngology residency programs offered no formal training in allergy. That situation had improved by 2006, when 62% of programs had active allergy programs, and the remainder were adding them.[1,2]

Allergic disease and sinusitis are among the most common medical conditions in the United States.[3] Ten to 20 percent of the population in western societies is affected, translating to 30 to 60 million annually in the United States alone. Immunoglobulin E (IgE)-mediated sensitivity to inhalant allergens is identifiable in 60% of patients with chronic rhinosinusitis. Allergy and/or sinusitis, affecting children and adults, account for significant morbidity and decrease in quality of life, increased direct medical costs, and indirect costs that include loss of productivity, absence from work or school, and poor performance when present.

But allergies and their effects are not limited to the nose. Food allergy is also an often-unrecognized clinical entity that has been implicated as a cause in many types of chronic inflammatory conditions. Chronic laryngitis, Meniere disease, asthma, sleep disorders, and eosinophilic esophagitis have been recognized as having an inhalant and/or dietary allergic component in some patients. When identified, treatment is targeted to the underlying allergy, resulting in significant patient benefit.

I congratulate Drs Ramanathan and Mims on putting together this comprehensive collection of pertinent articles encompassing the breadth of Otolaryngologic Allergy. The reader will be treated to an in-depth discussion of diagnostic techniques, including allergy testing, understanding of the nasal epithelium and the allergy-sinusitis relationship, extranasal manifestations of allergy, pharmacotherapy, and immunotherapy,

Otolaryngol Clin N Am 50 (2017) xv–xvi
https://doi.org/10.1016/j.otc.2017.09.022
0030-6665/17/© 2017 Published by Elsevier Inc.

both sublingual and subcutaneous, and how to handle anaphylaxis. The future of allergy treatment is very interesting, and otolaryngologists are poised at the crest of it.

The otolaryngologist–head and neck surgeon is uniquely qualified to perform comprehensive medical and surgical management for patients with complex disease processes involving a component of allergy. This issue of *Otolaryngologic Clinics of North America* enables the reader to formulate their own integrated approach to allergy within a busy otolaryngology practice, facilitating prompt diagnosis and optimizing treatment.

Sujana S. Chandrasekhar, MD
New York Otology
Hofstra-Northwell School of Medicine
Mount Sinai School of Medicine
210 East 64th Street, 3rd Floor
New York, NY 10065, USA

E-mail address:
ssc@nyotology.com

REFERENCES

1. Osguthorpe JD. Allergy and immunology training in otolaryngology residency programs. Arch Otolaryngol 1985;111(12):779–80.
2. Lin SY, Mabry RL. Allergy practice in the academic otolaryngology setting: results of a comprehensive survey. Otolaryngol Head Neck Surg 2006;134(1):25–7.
3. Seidman MD, Gurgel RK, Lin SY, et al. Clinical practice guideline: allergic rhinitis. Otolaryngol Head Neck Surg 2015;152(1 Suppl):S1–43.

Preface

Allergy for the Otolaryngologist

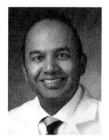
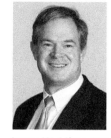

Murugappan (Murray) Ramanathan Jr, MD, FACS   James W. Mims, MD
Editors

The diagnosis and treatment of allergic disease is an integral part of otolaryngology practice, where care for inflammatory disorders of the nose, sinuses, and upper airway is common. This issue of *Otolaryngologic Clinics of North America* is designed to bring the practicing otolaryngologist up to date by focusing on where developments have occurred.

Drs Ramanathan and London discuss how the nasal and sinus epithelium acts as more than just a barrier and participates in the regulation and pathophysiology of nasal and sinus inflammation. While allergies are sometimes considered primarily in the context of allergic rhinitis by otolaryngologists, Drs Toskala, Shtraks, and Krouse provide compelling reasons that evaluation of the upper and lower respiratory track is the best practice, and they look at other associated diseases that affect allergic patients disproportionally. The relationship between chronic sinusitis and allergic rhinitis continues to be nuanced, and Drs Halderman and Tully provide a balanced review of the current literature of these two overlapping nasal inflammatory processes.

Ear symptoms and allergy continues to be a difficult topic with conflicting literature, and Drs Yang and Brook offer a thoughtful review of the studies available.

Current updates to allergy testing (Drs Platt and Wulu) are included, along with treatment advances focusing on sublingual therapy (Drs Roxbury, Lin, Edwards, and Wise) and the arrival of new monoclonal biologics (Drs Ghadersohi, Tan, Marino, and Luong). As more providers offer sublingual immunotherapy, the use of fewer allergens in treating polysensitized patients has become a pertinent clinical question. Dr Damask reviews the evidence on immunotherapy with fewer allergens.

Another large development in the management of allergy is the successful prevention of peanut allergy, as discussed by Dr Franzese, along with other food allergy updates.

Otolaryngol Clin N Am 50 (2017) xvii–xviii
https://doi.org/10.1016/j.otc.2017.09.019
0030-6665/17/© 2017 Published by Elsevier Inc.   **oto.theclinics.com**

Finally, Drs Marino and Luong share their perspective on future developments in the diagnosis and treatment of allergic disease. We believe this collection of articles provides the practicing otolaryngologist with a consolidated account of the recent developments in allergic disease.

We hope you find reading these articles as educational as we did.

Murugappan (Murray) Ramanathan Jr, MD, FACS
Director, National Capitol Region
Associate Professor
Rhinology and Endoscopic Skull Base Surgery
Departments of Otolaryngology Head and Neck Surgery and Neurosurgery
The Johns Hopkins University School of Medicine
601 N. Caroline Sreet JHOC 6263
Baltimore, MD 21287, USA

James W. Mims, MD
Department of Otolaryngology
Wake Forest Baptist Health
1 Medical Center Boulevard
Winston-Salem, NC 27157, USA

E-mail addresses:
mramana3@jhmi.edu (M. Ramanathan)
wmims@wakehealth.edu (J.W. Mims)

Advancements and Dilemmas in the Management of Allergy

James W. Mims, MD

KEYWORDS

- Allergy • Allergic rhinitis • Prevention • Allergy testing • Sublingual immunotherapy
- Desensitization

KEY POINTS

- Prevention of peanut allergy has been demonstrated through intentional oral exposure to peanut protein to promote tolerance.
- The diagnosis of inhalant allergy has not changed substantially, but continued research into component (or molecular) immunoglobulin E testing and research on local allergy may improve the accuracy of allergy testing in the future.
- Efficacious immunotherapy has expanded to include sublingual drops, sublingual tablets, and subcutaneous immunotherapy.
- With a wider variety of immunotherapy options, clinical decisions on allergen selection, such as the efficacy of sublingual tablets in polyallergic patients, have become more relevant.
- More humanized immunoglobulins targeting specific receptors and mediators of allergic inflammation (biologics) are now available, providing new options for patients with severe asthma and atopic conditions.

INTRODUCTION

The options for diagnosing and managing allergic disease have broadened over the last several years, creating new considerations for clinical allergists. This article provides a cursory synopsis of issues that have arisen in the literature and how clinical practitioners might alter their assessment and management of allergic patients.

PREVENTION

The prevalence of allergic rhinitis and other atopic conditions (specifically food allergies) has increased in the United States and other developed countries.[1] The

Department of Otolaryngology, Wake Forest School of Medicine, Medical Center Boulevard, Winston-Salem, NC 27157, USA
E-mail address: wmims@wakehealth.edu

Otolaryngol Clin N Am 50 (2017) 1037–1042
http://dx.doi.org/10.1016/j.otc.2017.08.001
0030-6665/17/Crown Copyright © 2017 Published by Elsevier Inc. All rights reserved.

reasons for this are not clear, and several theories have been offered including fewer childhood infections,[2,3] lower vitamin D levels,[4] changes in diets,[5] and exposures to a greater array of chemicals.[6] Studies that have tried to prevent inhalant allergic disease through decreased exposure to allergen sources such as dust mites or animal dander have often failed to show benefit or had conflicting results.[7,8]

The LEAP study advanced understanding by successfully preventing the development of peanut allergy in high-risk infants by intentional oral exposure to peanut proteins.[9] The paradigm shift of prevention through exposure to allergen rather than avoidance of allergen may lead to other successful prevention strategies that are certain to be investigated. The prevention of allergic rhinitis or allergic asthma has not been robustly demonstrated at this time.

DIAGNOSIS

The false-positive rate of sIgE testing (whether in sera or by skin testing) has been problematically high in the general population.[1] Fifty-four percent of the US population was skin prick test (SPT) positive per a Centers for Disease Control and Preventionsurvey.[10] As such, the clinical assessment of allergic rhinitis is central for making the correct diagnosis. Although the symptoms caused by intermittent and seasonal rhinitis, including itching, sneezing, rhinorrhea, and nasal congestion provide an identifiable pattern, the dominance of nasal congestion in perennial allergies has a broader differential diagnosis, including nonallergic rhinitis, mixed rhinitis, anatomic contributions, and chronic rhino-sinusitis. Clinically, selecting allergens for testing and knowing which positive tests are clinically relevant is challenging. Although major advances in the diagnosis of inhalant allergic disease have not gained wide-spread clinical use, there are some new technologies on the horizon.

Component or molecular diagnosis of allergy refers to delineating the IgE reactivity by the protein the allergen binds rather than the source material alone.[11,12] For example, component results for the dust mite *Dermatophagoides pteronyssinus* could be provided as Der p1 and Der p2. Potentially, component testing would better identify which allergens were more clinically important and identify cross-reactivity across different allergic sources.[11] However, the relationship between clinical allergic symptoms and component testing results may be complicated and require more research and population-specific data to be interpretable. Complex test results may lead to either computer-assisted interpretation of component testing or isolating a few clinical scenarios where certain component tests are clinically meaningful.

Local IgE in allergic rhinitis refers to presence of allergen-specific IgE in nasal secretions or tissues that can be detected when skin or sera-specific IgE testing is negative.[13-15] Standardized methods for collection and testing have not yet been established. If a standard method is agreed upon, identifying the clinical significance will remain a research goal. Adding to the confusion, nasal polyps also stain positive for polyclonal IgE; however, the relevance to specific allergic disease remains unclear, as the available literature shows that nasal polyposis and allergic rhinitis are not closely correlated.[16]

MANAGEMENT OF ALLERGIC DISEASE

For inhalant allergy, management of disease is classically discussed in terms of avoidance (or reduction of exposure through environmental control), pharmacotherapy, and immunotherapy.[1] Management with biologics, which refers to using humanized antibodies targeted against elements of the allergic inflammatory network, is also in use clinically.[17]

Avoidance

One of the main tenants of allergy therapy is education on what sources are causing an individual's symptoms and trying to reduce symptoms by limiting exposure. However, strategies to reduce symptoms through use of dehumidifiers, air filters, dust mite covers, pet washing, and other interventions have rarely shown a significant decrease in symptoms, although reduction of antigen is often demonstrated.[1] Reducing allergen exposure enough to reduce symptoms in an already sensitized individual seems to be difficult to achieve in most situations. Evidence-based counseling would suggest that resources would be better utilized on more proven management options.

Pharmacology

Nonsedating antihistamines and intranasal corticosteroid sprays are now over the counter in the United States. Still, professional medical providers remain the trusted source of information on how to best select medications to manage allergic symptoms. There are likely several areas where the use of medications for allergic rhinitis could be optimized. Four suggestions based on the literature stand out.

Oral forms of sedating antihistamines may be overused by the allergic population. Less-sedating and nonsedating antihistamines clearly have a better benefit/adverse effect profile and should be advocated in most situations.[1,18]

Studies show limited benefit of adding an oral antihistamine to an intranasal corticosteroid; however, this combination seems commonly utilized.[1,19,20] There may be specific cases where patient preference or poor symptom control with INCS alone make this combination reasonable.[21]

Montelukast has been identified as a poor first-line choice in allergic rhinitis and perhaps overprescribed for this indication in patients without asthma.[1]

Consideration of the high rate of concomitant allergic conjunctivitis with allergic rhinitis should influence pharmacologic choices more.[22]

For patients with severe disease, especially steroid-dependent asthma commonly encountered by otolaryngologists in aspirin exacerbated respiratory disease (AERD) and other chronic sinusitis with polyps patients, monoclonal antibodies targeting the workings of inflammatory mediators such as interleukin (IL-5) and IgE are available.[17] These seem especially suited for severe disease that is refractory to other measures due their expense and are further discussed in other articles in this issue.

Desensitization

The role of sublingual immunotherapy (SLIT) continues to be source of debate among allergy specialists.[23,24] Although multiple trials have shown efficacy,[24] the optimal regimen and dosage are not known.[25] There is also not a clear understanding of why some trials show efficacy, and others do not.[25]

SLIT is provided as sublingual drops prepared by allergy specialists and as commercially available tablets. Tablets are available for grass and ragweed, and a tablet for dust mite allergy was recently approved by the US Food and Drug Administration.

Many otolaryngologists employ sublingual therapy, and there seems to be enthusiasm from patients for a form of immunotherapy that does not require as many office visits, waiting periods, and needle sticks.

Traditionally, allergen-specific immunotherapy has targeted multiple allergens in the polyallergic patient. However, the scientific support for treating multiple allergens compared with fewer allergens is minimal.[26–28] In SLIT, effective doses may be 30 times higher the monthly totals used in subcutaneous immunotherapy.[25] Providers are faced with cost and logistical realities that have led to questions about whether fewer allergens can be used to treat polysensitized patients. Currently there is some scientific uncertainty about the relative efficacy between SLIT and subcutaneous immunotherapy, as well as uncertainty about the number of allergens to treat. The clinician's role now involves helping patients make an informed decision in selecting sublingual drops, sublingual tablets, or subcutaneous immunotherapy in terms of efficacy, time, costs, and convenience.

Another form of desensitization that has received in attention in the literature is aspirin desensitization. Research into AERD suggests a higher identification rate when aspirin challenges are employed with some advocating for a larger role of aspirin desensitization.[29] Despite newer biologics and aspirin desensitization, AERD patients remain difficult to manage.

Gene Therapy

In a recent animal study, gene therapy was successfully employed to silence the Th2 immune response to a specific allergen-provoked inflammation.[30] Gene therapy for allergic disease has not been demonstrated in people, and application in a clinical setting is not expected soon. However, the genetic understanding of allergic disease and the ability to manipulate genes continue to improve.

SUMMARY

The diagnosis and treatment of allergic disease continue to advance and challenge clinicians with increasing complexity and new opportunities. For decades, the foundation of treating severe inhalant allergies relied on skin testing and subcutaneous immunotherapy, but component testing, prevention through exposure, local allergy, biologics, and sublingual immunotherapy are among the advances that have entered the literature and are finding clinical application. The next generation of providers who treat allergic diseases will have new tools and treatment options, but also will face greater complexities. In addition to more research, mechanisms to deal with the increasing complexity may also need to coevolve.

REFERENCES

1. Seidman MD, Gurgel RK, Lin SY, et al. Clinical practice guideline: allergic rhinitis. Otolaryngol Head Neck Surg 2015;152:S1–43.
2. Strachan DP. Hay fever, hygiene, and household size. BMJ 1989;299:1259–60.
3. Daley D. The evolution of the hygiene hypothesis: the role of early-life exposures to viruses and microbes and their relationship to asthma and allergic diseases. Curr Opin Allergy Clin Immunol 2014;14:390–6.
4. Kim YH, Kim KW, Kim MJ, et al. Vitamin D levels in allergic rhinitis: a systematic review and meta-analysis. Pediatr Allergy Immunol 2016;27:580–90.
5. Saadeh D, Salameh P, Baldi I, et al. Diet and allergic diseases among population aged 0 to 18 years: myth or reality? Nutrients 2013;5:3399–423.
6. Baldacci S, Maio S, Cerrai S, et al. Allergy and asthma: Effects of the exposure to particulate matter and biological allergens. Respir Med 2015;109:1089–104.
7. Arshad SH, Bateman B, Matthews SM. Primary prevention of asthma and atopy during childhood by allergen avoidance in infancy: a randomised controlled study. Thorax 2003;58:489–93.
8. Custovic A, Simpson BM, Simpson A, et al. Effect of environmental manipulation in pregnancy and early life on respiratory symptoms and atopy during first year of life: a randomised trial. Lancet 2001;358:188–93.

9. Du Toit G, Roberts G, Sayre PH, et al. Randomized trial of peanut consumption in infants at risk for peanut allergy. N Engl J Med 2015;372:803–13.

10. Arbes SJ Jr, Gergen PJ, Elliott L, et al. Prevalences of positive skin test responses to 10 common allergens in the US population: results from the third National Health and Nutrition Examination Survey. J Allergy Clin Immunol 2005;116: 377–83.

11. Ciprandi G, Incorvaia C, Frati F, Italian Study Group on Polysensitization. Management of polysensitized patient: from molecular diagnostics to biomolecular immunotherapy. Expert Rev Clin Immunol 2015;11:973–6.

12. Matricardi PM, Kleine-Tebbe J, Hoffmann HJ, et al. EAACI molecular allergology user's guide. Pediatr Allergy Immunol 2016;27(Suppl 23):1–250.

13. Cheng KJ, Zhou ML, Xu YY, et al. The role of local allergy in the nasal inflammation. Eur Arch Otorhinolaryngol 2017;274(9):3275–81.

14. Reisacher WR, Suurna MV, Rochlin K, et al. Oral mucosal immunotherapy for allergic rhinitis: A pilot study. Allergy Rhinol (Providence) 2016;7:21–8.

15. Wise SK, Ahn CN, Schlosser RJ. Localized immunoglobulin E expression in allergic rhinitis and nasal polyposis. Curr Opin Otolaryngol Head Neck Surg 2009;17:216–22.

16. Orlandi RR, Kingdom TT, Hwang PH, et al. International consensus statement on allergy and rhinology: rhinosinusitis. Int Forum Allergy Rhinol 2016;6(Suppl 1): S22–209.

17. Lam K, Kern RC, Luong A. Is there a future for biologics in the management of chronic rhinosinusitis? Int Forum Allergy Rhinol 2016;6:935–42.

18. Church MK, Maurer M, Simons FE, et al. Risk of first-generation H(1)-antihistamines: a GA(2)LEN position paper. Allergy 2010;65:459–66.

19. Anolik R, Mometasone Furoate Nasal Spray With Loratadine Study Group. Clinical benefits of combination treatment with mometasone furoate nasal spray and loratadine vs monotherapy with mometasone furoate in the treatment of seasonal allergic rhinitis. Ann Allergy Asthma Immunol 2008;100:264–71.

20. Di Lorenzo G, Pacor ML, Pellitteri ME, et al. Randomized placebo-controlled trial comparing fluticasone aqueous nasal spray in mono-therapy, fluticasone plus cetirizine, fluticasone plus montelukast and cetirizine plus montelukast for seasonal allergic rhinitis. Clin Exp Allergy 2004;34:259–67.

21. Brozek JL, Bousquet J, Agache I, et al. Allergic Rhinitis and its Impact on Asthma (ARIA) guidelines-2016 revision. J Allergy Clin Immunol 2017. [Epub ahead of print].

22. Cingi C, Gevaert P, Mosges R, et al. Multi-morbidities of allergic rhinitis in adults: European Academy of Allergy and Clinical Immunology Task Force report. Clin Transl Allergy 2017;7:17.

23. Greenhawt M, Oppenheimer J, Nelson M, et al. Sublingual immunotherapy: a focused allergen immunotherapy practice parameter update. Ann Allergy Asthma Immunol 2017;118:276–82.e272.

24. Lin SY, Erekosima N, Kim JM, et al. Sublingual immunotherapy for the treatment of allergic rhinoconjunctivitis and asthma: a systematic review. JAMA 2013;309: 1278–88.

25. Leatherman BD, Khalid A, Lee S, et al. Dosing of sublingual immunotherapy for allergic rhinitis: evidence-based review with recommendations. Int Forum Allergy Rhinol 2015;5:773–83.

26. Lowell FC, Franklin W. A double-blind study of the effectiveness and specificity of injecton therapy in ragweed hay fever. N Engl J Med 1965;273:675–9.

27. Franklin W, Lowell FC. Comparison of two dosages of ragweed extract in the treatment of pollenosis. JAMA 1967;201:915–7.
28. Nelson HS. Multiallergen immunotherapy for allergic rhinitis and asthma. J Allergy Clin Immunol 2009;123:763–9.
29. Stevenson DD, White AA. Clinical characteristics of aspirin-exacerbated respiratory disease. Immunol Allergy Clin N Am 2016;36:643–55.
30. Al-Kouba J, Wilkinson AN, Starkey MR, et al. Allergen-encoding bone marrow transfer inactivates allergic T cell responses, alleviating airway inflammation. JCI Insight 2017;2 [pii:85742].

The Role of the Sinonasal Epithelium in Allergic Rhinitis

Nyall R. London Jr, MD, PhD, Murugappan Ramanathan Jr, MD*

KEYWORDS

- Allergic rhinitis • Epithelial permeability • House dust mite
- Sinonasal barrier dysfunction • Tight junctions

KEY POINTS

- The sinonasal epithelial barrier is at the interface between the external airborne environment and the underlying tissue. This barrier is comprised of tight junction and adherens junction proteins.
- Barrier dysfunction has been hypothesized to contribute to allergic disease such as allergic rhinitis through increased passage of antigens and exposure of underlying tissue to these stimuli.
- Mechanisms of sinonasal epithelial barrier disruption may include antigen proteolytic activity, inflammatory cytokine-mediated tight junction breakdown, or exacerbation from environmental stimuli such as particulate matter or diesel exhaust.
- Mechanisms of sinonasal epithelial barrier stabilization include corticosteroids and nuclear erythroid 2-related factor 2 (Nrf2) cytoprotective pathway activation.
- Future studies will help to elucidate the importance of barrier disruption in allergic rhinitis (AR) and whether barrier stabilization may improve AR pathophysiology.

INTRODUCTION

The sinonasal airway is at the gateway between the external airborne environment and the human body. As an initial contact point during inhalation, the sinonasal airway serves multiple roles including thermoregulation, moisturization, removal of airborne particles, and response to infectious agents.[1] Infectious airborne stimuli are combatted by innate immune mechanisms including mucociliary clearance, bitter taste receptors, sinonasal epithelial barrier function, and innate immune effector cells.[2–4]

The sinonasal airway is bombarded on a daily basis with a host of noxious stimuli, some of which may be allergenic. An allergic response to inhaled stimuli can cause an immunoglobulin E (IgE)-mediated inflammatory response characterized by symptoms

Disclosure Statement: The authors declare no relevant conflicts of interest.
Department of Otolaryngology–Head and Neck Surgery, Johns Hopkins, Baltimore, MD, USA
* Corresponding author. 601 North Caroline Street, 6th Floor, Baltimore, MD 21287.
E-mail address: mramana3@jhmi.edu

Otolaryngol Clin N Am 50 (2017) 1043–1050
http://dx.doi.org/10.1016/j.otc.2017.08.002
0030-6665/17/© 2017 Elsevier Inc. All rights reserved.

including rhinorrhea, nasal itching, sneezing, and congestion.[5] This response is known as allergic rhinitis (AR) and is among the most common human ailments. Indeed, the prevalence of AR has been estimated to be 10% to 20% in the United States.[6] A diagnosis of AR is obtained by patient history, confirmation of an IgE-mediated mechanism through skin prick or serum testing, and an allergic response to the known trigger.[7] Allergic rhinitis is classified based on the temporal exposure of the allergenic trigger as seasonal, episodic, or perennial, as well as by the frequency and severity of symptoms.[5] Common known triggers include antigens such as dust mite, pollen, grass, tree, and pets. Current empiric therapeutic strategies include intranasal steroids, antihistamines, and exposure control. Those patients who do not have an adequate response may also consider immunotherapy as an effective treatment option.[5,8]

There has been significant interest in the role the sinonasal epithelial barrier plays in sinonasal disease such as AR (**Fig. 1**).[2,9,10] This barrier is created between sinonasal epithelial cells via apical transmembrane and scaffold protein interactions including tight junction proteins such as zonula occludens-1 (ZO-1), claudin family members, occludin, and junctional adhesion molecule-A (JAM-A). Adherens junction proteins such as epithelial cadherin (E-cadherin) create intercellular interactions. Together, these junction proteins function to limit intercellular passage of fluid and protect the underlying tissue from exposure to noxious and allergenic stimuli. Dysfunction of epithelial barrier function has been hypothesized to contribute to allergic disease through allowing increased passage of antigens and exposure of underlying tissue to these stimuli. The purpose of this article is to investigate the current understanding of the role of the sinonasal epithelial barrier in allergic rhinitis.

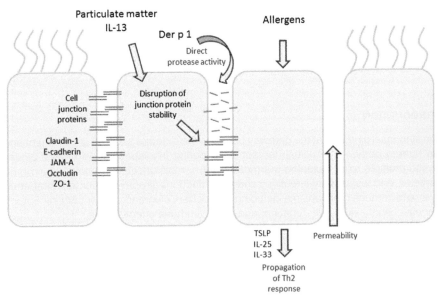

Fig. 1. The sinonasal barrier is comprised of a variety of tight and adherens cell junction proteins. Destabilization of these protein interactions occurs via direct proteolysis or through stimulation of intracellular signaling mechanisms, resulting in increased epithelial permeability. The sinonasal epithelium also secretes inflammatory cytokines including TSLP, IL-25, and IL-33, which propagate additional inflammatory pathways and Th2-mediated inflammation. (*From* Woodworth BA, Poetker DM, Reh DD (eds): Rhinosinusitis with Nasal Polyposis. Adv Otorhinolaryngol. Basel, Karger, 2016;79:70; with permission.)

EPITHELIAL BARRIER FUNCTION IN ATOPIC DISEASE

Epithelial barrier dysfunction has been linked to chronic inflammatory disease of multiple organ systems including atopic dermatitis, inflammatory bowel disease, asthma, and chronic rhinosinusitis (CRS). For example, single nucleotide polymorphisms in claudin-1, protocadherin-1, and E-cadherin have been linked to atopic dermatitis, asthma, and Crohn disease.[11–13] Decreased claudin-18 expression has been reported in asthmatic patients, and claudin-18 knockout mice demonstrate significantly increased airway responsiveness following intranasal aspergillus sensitization.[14] Decreased barrier function and decreased expression of ZO-1, claudin-1, and occludin have been noted in biopsy specimens from patients with CRS with nasal polyps.[15,16] Thus epithelial barrier dysfunction has been linked to chronic inflammatory disease through multiple lines of evidence.

Screening studies using microarray gene expression, RNA-seq, and nasal mucus proteomics have suggested a role for barrier dysfunction in AR.[17–19] These findings are supported by multiple studies reporting decreased sinonasal epithelial cell junction protein expression in allergic rhinitis. Lee and colleagues[20] reported decreased ZO-1 and E-cadherin expression in the nasal epithelium of patients with AR. Consistent with these findings, Steelant and colleagues[21] reported decreased ZO-1 and occludin expression as assessed by RT-qPCR and weak immunofluorescent staining in AR biopsy specimens.

Steelant and colleagues[21] have also investigated the functional consequences of barrier dysfunction in symptomatic AR. To do so, they first obtained nasal biopsy specimens from control and house dust mite (HDM)-AR patients. These ex vivo mucosal explants were placed in an Ussing chamber, which measures transtissue electrical resistance as a measurement of epithelial barrier function. Nasal mucosa explants from HDM-AR patients were found to have a statistically significant decrease in transtissue resistance, indicating disrupted barrier function compared with control specimens.[21] As a means to assess epithelial barrier dysfunction to macromolecules, fluorescein isothiocyanate-dextran 4 kDa (FD4) transit across ex vivo mucosal explants was also tested. This demonstrated an approximately twofold increase of FD4 leak across HDM-AR specimens compared with controls.[21] Lastly, the visual analog scale correlated inversely with major symptoms in HDM-AR but not controls.

In addition to these ex vivo results, in vitro studies have also been suggestive of barrier disruption in AR. Nasal epithelial cells isolated from inferior turbinates and grown on an air liquid interface in culture for 21 days demonstrated a baseline decrease in barrier function as demonstrated by transepithelial electrical resistance (TEER) and FD4 transit compared with control samples. Furthermore, these cells grown in culture demonstrated decreased expression of ZO-1 and occludin as assessed by RT-qPCR and immunofluorescence.[21] Lee and colleagues[20] reported decreased E-cadherin expression in cultured cells from AR compared with control stimulated with interleukin-4 (IL-4), IL-5, and tumor necrosis factor-alpha (TNF-α). Collectively, these results suggest that permanent changes in barrier function occur to sinonasal epithelial cells in AR perpetuated in culture.

DISRUPTION OF BARRIER FUNCTION IN ALLERGIC RHINITIS MAY OCCUR THROUGH MULTIPLE MECHANISMS

Mechanisms of sinonasal barrier disruption have been described including allergen proteolytic activity and inflammatory cytokine-mediated disruption. One well-described example of proteolytic activity is the HDM cysteine proteinase antigen

Der p 1.[22] Der p 1 has been reported to cleave extracellular domain sites in occludin and in claudin-1, resulting in increased epithelial permeability and Der p 1 transit through the epithelial barrier.[22] Furthermore, Der p 1 has been shown to cause a time-dependent breakdown of tight junctions as well as ZO-1 mislocalization from tight junctions.[23] Inhibition of the protease activity of Der p 1 as a therapeutic strategy for reducing HDM-induced barrier dysfunction has been reported.[24]

Multiple inflammatory cytokines have been implicated in AR pathogenesis including IL-33, an IL-1-like cytokine constitutively expressed in the nucleus of nasal epithelial cells. Upon secretion from nasal epithelial cells, IL-33 is known to incite a Th2 response. Increased IL-33 expression has been found in the serum of AR patients and a single nucleotide polymorphism (SNP) association reported in IL-33 and AR.[25] In order to test the necessity of IL-33 in AR pathogenesis, Haenuki and colleagues[26] developed IL-33 knockout mice and a ragweed murine model of AR in which mice are subjected to intranasal instillation of ragweed pollen after intraperitoneal sensitization. Using the ragweed model, IL-33 knockout mice demonstrated decreased eosinophil accumulation, decreased ability to mount an IgE response, and decreased cytokine expression IL-4, IL-5, and IL-13 compared with controls.[26] These effects in IL-33 knockout mice were reversed when IL-33 knockout mice were exposed to ragweed pollen and recombinant IL-33.[26]

IL-33 has been demonstrated to act on type 2 innate lymphoid cells (ILC2s), which in turn have recently been reported to disrupt bronchial epithelial barrier integrity through IL-13 release.[27] In this study, human bronchial epithelial cells were grown at an air liquid interface, and ILC2s were applied basolaterally. A significant disruption in epithelial barrier function was evidenced by decreased transepithelial electrical resistance and increased FITC-dextran leak.[27] Although IL-33 administration alone was not sufficient to disrupt barrier function, IL-33 administration in combination with ILC2s led to a significant exacerbation of ILC2-mediated leak. Decreased barrier integrity was significantly improved with anti-IL-13 treatment, suggesting an IL-13-dependent mechanism. Interestingly, intranasal administration of IL-33 in control but not ILC2 deficient mice increased barrier disruption as assessed by α2-macroglobulin and transferrin in bronchoalveolar lavage samples.[27] Occludin and ZO-1 expression was also disrupted by IL-33 administration as measured by decreased immunofluorescence and mRNA expression in control but not ILC2 deficient mice.[27] Lastly, in vivo intranasal administration of IL-13 was sufficient to disrupt bronchial epithelial cell integrity as evidenced by increased α2-macroglobulin and transferrin levels in bronchoalveolar lavage fluid.

PARTICULATE MATTER MAY EXACERBATE ALLERGIC RHINITIS IN ANIMAL MODELS

Another potential mechanism of sinonasal barrier breakdown and subsequent exacerbation of atopic disease is via particulate matter (PM) exposure. Indeed, the documented harmful effects of PM on human health are pervasive and include cardiovascular disease, aggravation of chronic respiratory disease, and premature death.[28] Particulate matter contains redox-active chemicals and transition metals and may exert its disruptive effects through the generation of reactive oxygen species.[29] To test whether PM can cause sinonasal epithelial barrier dysfunction in vitro, sinonasal epithelial cells grown at an air-liquid interface were exposed to PM. Four hours after exposure, there was a significant decrease in barrier function as assessed by a reduction in TEER and increased paracellular flux of FD4.[29] Furthermore, the cell surface localization of ZO-1, JAM-A, and occludin was found to be reduced after PM exposure as assessed by immunofluorescence.[29]

To test the effects of inhalation of airborne fine particulate matter, mice were exposed to concentrated particulate matter for 16 weeks. The concentration used was approximately 60 µg per cubic meter, which is lower than that reported in some major global cities.[30] Using this in vivo model, a significant increase in serum albumin accumulation in nasal lavage fluid was observed, indicative of barrier dysfunction.[30] Furthermore, immunofluorescence against E-cadherin and claudin-1 in sinonasal mucosa of mice exposed to concentrated PM demonstrated decreased E-cadherin and claudin-1 expression. In addition to barrier disruption, a significant increase in inflammation was reported including macrophage, neutrophil, and eosinophil accumulation, as well as increased expression of IL-13 and eotaxin-1.[30] Although the exact mechanism of action has yet to be determined, these observational studies demonstrate that chronic inhalation of PM in vivo is sufficient to cause nonallergic eosinophilic inflammation.

To determine whether inhaled pollutants may exacerbate AR in vivo, Fukuoka and colleagues[31] pretreated mice with intranasal diesel exhaust particles (DEPs) prior to ragweed pollen challenge. They observed increased sneezing after DEP pretreatment compared with controls, indicative of exacerbation of AR symptoms. DEP treatment was found to disrupt ZO-1 expression in nasal mucosa in vivo as well as in RPMI 2650 cells in vitro. Lastly, antioxidant treatment inhibited DEP-induced epithelial junction disruption and sneezing exacerbation, suggestive of an oxidative stress mechanism of action for DEP.[31]

STABILIZING THE EPITHELIAL BARRIER

As there is evidence that epithelial barrier disruption contributes to AR, one may hypothesize that stabilizing the epithelial barrier may improve AR. Using the nasal explant system, Steelant and colleagues[21] reported that HDM-AR patients who used intranasal steroids were found to have significantly higher transepithelial electrical resistance and decreased flux of FD4 across the epithelial barrier. Furthermore, these explants had a higher expression of ZO-1 and occludin than control. Interestingly, when nasal epithelial cells were cultured in vitro at an air-liquid interface, fluticasone treatment alone significantly improved epithelial barrier function as assessed by TEER and FD4 paracellular flux.[21] Fluticasone treatment also increased expression of ZO-1 and occludin.[21] Furthermore, fluticasone pretreatment reduced IL-4-induced epithelial barrier dysfunction. Lastly, the improved baseline barrier function with fluticasone was negated in vitro by pretreatment with a glucocorticoid receptor antagonist.[21] Thus glucocorticoids may stabilize sinonasal epithelial barrier function.

One potential target for stabilization of the epithelial barrier is the nuclear erythroid 2-related factor 2 (Nrf2) cytoprotective pathway. Upon activation, Nrf2 translocates to the nucleus and increases expression of cytoprotective genes.[29] One known activator of the Nrf2 pathway is the small molecule sulforaphane (SFN). Sinonasal epithelial cells pretreated with SFN had significantly reduced PM-mediated barrier disruption as assessed by TEER and FITC-dextran leak.[29] Furthermore, SFN pretreatment decreased PM-mediated disruption of ZO-1, JAM-A, and claudin-1 in vitro. In a similar manner, SFN has been reported to improve cigarette smoke extract and HDM-induced disruption of sinonasal epithelial barrier function and ZO-1 expression.[32,33] Future in vivo studies will help to elucidate the importance of the Nrf2 pathway in vivo.

PROPAGATION OF TH2 INFLAMMATION BY EPITHELIAL-DERIVED CYTOKINES

The sinonasal epithelium also acts to exacerbate AR through secretion of inflammatory cytokines including thymic stromal lymphopoietin (TSLP), IL-25, and IL-33.[34]

These cytokines act on surrounding cells including ILC2s which in turn secrete IL-4, IL-5, and IL-13.[2] These downstream cytokines act to instigate a Th2-mediated response and recruit additional inflammatory cells such as eosinophils. Broad neutralization of these downstream cytokines has been reported to significantly reduce eosinophil accumulation and plasma protein exudates in a murine ovalbumin model of AR.[35] Furthermore, ILC2s may interact directly with T cells to stimulate T cell activation.[2,36] Thus epithelial-derived cytokines may instigate a chain reaction of signaling pathways, contributing to the pathogenesis of AR.

The importance of sinonasal epithelial-derived cytokines has been investigated in murine acute and chronic models of allergic rhinitis. One study found decreased Th2 activation (as assessed by increased IL-4, IL-5, and IL-13 production) and nasal eosinophilia in IL-33$^{-/-}$ mice when ragweed pollen was administered intranasally in an acute but not chronic model of AR.[37] Interestingly, while TSLP receptor (TSLPR)-deficient mice did not demonstrate a significant reduction in Th2 activation and nasal eosinophilia in the ragweed model, a significant decrease in serum ragweed-specific IgE levels and sneezing response was observed.[37] In a murine model of chronic rhinosinusitis with nasal polyposis characterized by chronic ovalbumin exposure combined with staphylococcal enterotoxin B, neutralization of IL-25 significantly reduced eosinophil accumulation and nasal polyp formation. Thus TSLP, IL-25, and IL-33 may be necessary for propagating differing aspects of Th2-mediated inflammation in allergen-mediated sinonasal inflammation.[38]

SUMMARY

The sinonasal airway is at the gateway between the external airborne environment and the human body. Epithelial barrier dysfunction has been linked to chronic inflammatory disease of multiple organ systems including atopic dermatitis, inflammatory bowel disease, asthma, and CRS. Disruption of epithelial barrier function has been hypothesized to contribute to allergic disease such as AR through increased passage of antigens and exposure of underlying tissue to these stimuli. Mechanisms of epithelial barrier destabilization presented here include proteolytic activity of the HDM Der p 1, IL-33 interplay with ILC2s to increase IL-13 expression, and exacerbation with PM or DEP. Future studies will help to understand the importance of barrier disruption in AR and whether barrier stabilization may improve AR pathophysiology.

REFERENCES

1. Beule AG. Physiology and pathophysiology of respiratory mucosa of the nose and the paranasal sinuses. GMS Curr Top Otorhinolaryngol Head Neck Surg 2010;9:Doc07.
2. London NR, Lane AP. Innate immunity and chronic rhinosinusitis: what we have learned from animal models. Laryngoscope Investig Otolaryngol 2016;1(3): 49–56.
3. Lee RJ, Kofonow JM, Rosen PL, et al. Bitter and sweet taste receptors regulate human upper respiratory innate immunity. J Clin Invest 2014;124(3):1393–405.
4. Carey RM, Workman AD, Chen B, et al. *Staphylococcus aureus* triggers nitric oxide production in human upper airway epithelium. Int Forum Allergy Rhinol 2015; 5(9):808–13.
5. Seidmen MD, Gurgel RK, Lin SY, et al. Clinical practice guideline: allergic rhinitis. Otolaryngol Head Neck Surg 2015;152(1S):S1–43.
6. Mims JW. Epidemiology of allergic rhinitis. Int Forum Allergy Rhinol 2014;4(Suppl 2): S18–20.

7. Hellings PW, Fokkens WJ, Bachert C, et al. Positioning the principles of precision medicine in care pathways for allergic rhinitis and chronic rhinosinusitis - an EUFOREA-ARIA-EPOS-AIRWAYS ICP statement. Allergy 2017;72(9):1297–305.

8. Lin SY, Erekosima N, Kim JM, et al. Sublingual immunotherapy for the treatment of allergic rhinoconjunctivitis and asthma: a systematic review. JAMA 2013;309(12): 1278–88.

9. London NR, Tharakan A, Ramanathan M. The role of innate immunity and aeroallergens in chronic rhinosinusitis. Adv Otorhinolaryngol 2016;79:69–77.

10. Steelant B, Seys SF, Boeckxstaens G, et al. Restoring airway epithelial barrier dysfunction: a new therapeutic challenge in allergic airway disease. Rhinology 2016;54(3):195–205.

11. De Benedetto A, Rafaels NM, McGirt LY, et al. Tight junction defects in patients with atopic dermatitis. J Allergy Clin Immunol 2011;127(3):773–86.

12. Mortensen LJ, Kreiner-Møller E, Hakonarson H, et al. The PCDH1 gene and asthma in early childhood. Eur Respir J 2014;43(3):792–800.

13. Muise AM, Walters TD, Glowacka WK, et al. Polymorphisms in E-cadherin (CDH1) result in a mis-localised cytoplasmic protein that is associated with Crohn's disease. Gut 2009;58(8):1121–7.

14. Sweerus K, Lachowicz-Scroggins M, Gordon E, et al. Claudin-18 deficiency is associated with airway epithelial barrier dysfunction and asthma. J Allergy Clin Immunol 2017;139(1):72–81.

15. Rogers GA, Den Beste K, Parkos CA, et al. Epithelial tight junction alterations in nasal polyposis. Int Forum Allergy Rhinol 2011;1(1):50–4.

16. Soyka MB, Wawrzyniak P, Eiwegger T, et al. Defective epithelial barrier in chronic rhinosinusitis: the regulation of tight junctions by IFN-γ and IL-4. J Allergy Clin Immunol 2012;130(5):1087–96.

17. Wagener AH, Zwinderman AH, Luiten S, et al. The impact of allergic rhinitis and asthma on human nasal and bronchial epithelial gene expression. PLoS One 2013;8(11):e80257.

18. Tomazic PV, Birner-Gruenberger R, Leitner A, et al. Nasal mucus proteomic changes reflect altered immune responses and epithelial permeability in patients with allergic rhinitis. J Allergy Clin Immunol 2014;133(3):741–50.

19. Ahuja SK, Manoharan MS, Harper NL, et al. Preservation of epithelial cell barrier function and muted inflammation in resistance to allergic rhinoconjunctivitis from house dust mite challenge. J Allergy Clin Immunol 2017;139(3):844–54.

20. Lee HJ, Kim B, Im NR, et al. Decreased expression of E-cadherin and ZO-1 in the nasal mucosa of patients with allergic rhinitis: altered regulation of E-cadherin by IL-4, IL-5, and TNF-alpha. Am J Rhinol Allergy 2016;30(3):173–8.

21. Steelant B, Farré R, Wawrzyniak P, et al. Impaired barrier function in patients with house dust mite-induced allergic rhinitis is accompanied by decreased occludin and zonula occludens-1 expression. J Allergy Clin Immunol 2016;137(4): 1043–53.

22. Wan H, Winton HL, Soeller C, et al. Der p 1 facilitates transepithelial allergen delivery by disruption of tight junctions. J Clin Invest 1999;104(1):123–33.

23. Wan H, Winton HL, Soeller C, et al. Quantitative structural and biochemical analyses of tight junction dynamics following exposure of epithelial cells to house dust mite allergen Der p 1. Clin Exp Allergy 2000;30(5):685–98.

24. John RJ, Rusznak C, Ramjee M, et al. Functional effects of the inhibition of the cysteine protease activity of the major house dust mite allergen Der p 1 by a novel peptide-based inhibitor. Clin Exp Allergy 2000;30(6):784–93.

25. Sakashita M, Yoshimoto T, Hirota T, et al. Association of serum interleukin-33 level and the interleukin-33 genetic variant with Japanese cedar pollinosis. Clin Exp Allergy 2008;38(12):1875–81.

26. Haenuki Y, Matsushita K, Futatsugi-Yumikura S, et al. A critical role of IL-33 in experimental allergic rhinitis. J Allergy Clin Immunol 2012;130(1):184–94.

27. Sugita K, Steer CA, Martinez-Gonzalez I, et al. Type 2 innate lymphoid cells disrupt bronchial epithelial barrier integrity by targeting tight junctions through IL-13 in asthmatic patients. J Allergy Clin Immunol 2017 [pii:S0091-6749(17) 30572-9/doi: 10.1016/j.jaci.2017.02.038].

28. Kim KH, Kabir E, Kabir S. A review on the human health impact of airborne particulate matter. Environ Int 2015;74:136–43.

29. London NR, Tharakan A, Rule AM, et al. Air pollutant-mediated disruption of sino-nasal epithelial cell barrier function is reversed by activation of the Nrf2 pathway. J Allergy Clin Immunol 2016;138(6):1736–8.

30. Ramanathan M, London NR Jr, Tharakan A, et al. Airborne particulate matter induces non-allergic eosinophilic sinonasal inflammation in mice. Am J Respir Cell Mol Biol 2017;57(1):59–65.

31. Fukuoka A, Matsushita K, Morikawa T, et al. Diesel exhaust particles exacerbate allergic rhinitis in mice by disrupting the nasal epithelial barrier. Clin Exp Allergy 2016;46(1):142–52.

32. Tharakan A, Halderman AA, Lane AP, et al. Reversal of cigarette smoke extract-induced sinonasal epithelial cell barrier dysfunction through Nrf2 activation. Int Forum Allergy Rhinol 2016;6(11):1145–50.

33. London NR, Tharakan A, Lane AP, et al. Nuclear erythroid 2-related factor 2 activation inhibits house dust mite-induced sinonasal epithelial cell barrier dysfunction. Int Forum Allergy Rhinol 2017;7(5):536–41.

34. Divekar R, Kita H. Recent advances in epithelium-derived cytokines (IL-33, IL-25, and thymic stromal lymphopoietin) and allergic inflammation. Curr Opin Allergy Clin Immunol 2015;15(1):98–103.

35. Sanden C, Mori M, Jogdand P, et al. Broad Th2 neutralization and anti-inflammatory action of pentosane polysulfate sodium in experimental allergic rhinitis. Immun Inflamm Dis 2017;5(3):300–9.

36. Vreugde S, Wormald PJ. Innate lymphoid type 2 cells in chronic rhinosinusitis. Curr Opin Allergy Clin Immunol 2016;16(1):7–12.

37. Akasaki S, Matsushita K, Kato Y, et al. Murine allergic rhinitis and nasal Th2 activation are mediated via TSLP- and IL-33-signaling pathways. Int Immunol 2016; 28(2):65–76.

38. Shin HW, Kim DK, Park MH, et al. IL-25 as a novel therapeutic target in nasal polyps of patients with chronic rhinosinusitis. J Allergy Clin Immunol 2015; 135(6):1476–85.

Manifestations of Inhalant Allergies Beyond the Nose

Julie P. Shtraks, MD, Elina Toskala, MD, PhD, MBA*

KEYWORDS

- Allergic rhinitis • Rhinosinusitis • Asthma • Laryngitis • Conjunctivitis
- Unified airway • United airway disease

KEY POINTS

- Allergic rhinitis, rhinosinusitis, and asthma frequently occur in the same patients.
- The upper and lower airways are linked both epidemiologically and pathophysiologically.
- Allergic rhinitis is a risk factor for the development of asthma, and treatment of rhinitis has been shown to improve asthma outcomes.
- Rhinosinusitis and asthma are linked, and comorbid sinusitis and asthma is associated with more severe clinical presentation.
- Allergic laryngitis is less well-understood; however, there is evidence of an epidemiologic link.

INTRODUCTION

Allergic inflammation affects both the upper and lower airways. The relationship between allergic rhinitis and its comorbidities, including chronic rhinosinusitis (CRS) and asthma, has been well-established. Given that a large part of the otolaryngologist's practice involves the diagnosis and management of upper airway disease, including allergic rhinitis, sinusitis, and laryngitis, knowledge of the manifestations of inhalant allergies beyond the nose is critical. The otolaryngologist may be the first physician to suspect and diagnose asthma in this at-risk patient population. As otolaryngologists, we therefore must be knowledgeable regarding the signs and symptoms of lower airway disease to ensure timely diagnosis of asthma and to optimize treatment of both upper and lower airway inflammatory diseases. A thorough understanding of the close relationship between allergic rhinitis, CRS, and asthma will facilitate early identification of asthma and improve patient outcomes.[1]

Department of Otolaryngology–Head and Neck Surgery, Lewis Katz School of Medicine at Temple University, 3440 North Broad Street, Kresge West 312, Philadelphia, PA 19140, USA
* Corresponding author.
E-mail address: Elina.toskala@tuhs.temple.edu

Otolaryngol Clin N Am 50 (2017) 1051–1064
http://dx.doi.org/10.1016/j.otc.2017.08.004
0030-6665/17/© 2017 Elsevier Inc. All rights reserved.

oto.theclinics.com

THE UNIFIED AIRWAY

The "unified airway" or "united airway disease" describes the concept of viewing the upper and lower airways as a single, functional unit. This model originated from the observation that allergic inflammation in response to an allergen is not confined to a specific organ, but rather it affects the entire respiratory tract. The nose, paranasal sinuses, pharynx, larynx, trachea, and bronchi through the pulmonary alveoli are included in this unit. Upon allergen exposure, local inflammatory processes occur along with a systemic response produced by the migration of proinflammatory mediators through the circulatory system. Under this model, upper and lower airway disease, including rhinitis, sinusitis, and asthma, can be thought of as different manifestations of the same disease.[2]

The upper and lower respiratory tracts share histologic structures in common, including pseudostratified columnar epithelium, basement membrane, lamina propria, and goblet cells. It follows that inflammatory processes are similar along the length of the respiratory tract. However, there are several structural differences that contribute to the unique physical manifestations of allergic inflammation in distinct respiratory sites; upper airway mucosa is richly vascular, whereas lower airway bronchial mucosa is characterized by the presence of smooth muscle. Inflammation of the nasal mucosa results in vasodilation and edema, whereas inflammation of the bronchial mucosa produces smooth muscle contraction.[3] The pathophysiologic link between the upper and lower airway has been demonstrated in several studies.[4–6] Stimulation with antigen at 1 respiratory site has been shown to produce an inflammatory response at distant and distinct respiratory sites. This "inflammatory cross-talk" supports the shared immunity mechanism to explain the unified airway.

Because the inflammation associated with allergy acts both locally and systemically, upper and lower airway pathology frequently coexist. Allergic rhinitis is the most common atopic disease. Not only is allergic rhinitis associated with asthma, but the presence of allergic rhinitis itself is considered a risk factor for the development of asthma. Long-term studies have demonstrated that allergic rhinitis is a risk factor for the future development of bronchial hyperresponsiveness and/or asthma. The risk of development of asthma is 3 times higher in patients with allergic or nonallergic rhinitis.[7] Patients with clinically severe sinonasal symptoms are at even greater risk for the development of asthma.[8] The prevalence of asthma in patients with rhinitis has been estimated to be as high as 40%, and approximately 80% of patients with asthma also have rhinitis. Furthermore, 30% of patients with allergic rhinitis who do not have asthma demonstrate bronchial hyperresponsiveness to methacholine or histamine challenge.[3] This supports the idea of "one airway, one disease."

The clinical impact of the unified airway has also been explored. Examination of prescription data revealed that patients with both asthma and allergic rhinitis had a higher percentage of prescription medication use than those with asthma alone.[1] Several studies have shown that treatment of rhinitis in patients with asthma produces clinical benefit in terms of reduction of lower airway symptoms, emergency room visits, and hospitalizations.[9–11]

RHINITIS AND ASTHMA
Epidemiologic Relationship and Clinical Implications

Allergic rhinitis is defined as symptomatic, immunoglobulin E (IgE)-mediated inflammation of the nasal mucosa after allergen exposure. Symptoms of allergic rhinitis include rhinorrhea, nasal congestion, obstruction, pruritus, and sneezing.[12] Asthma is a chronic respiratory disorder characterized by wheezing, coughing, chest tightness, and shortness of breath.[13] The epidemiologic relationship between rhinitis and asthma has been well-studied over the past several decades. Patients with allergic or nonallergic rhinitis are more likely to develop asthma than the average individual, and those with asthma are far more likely to suffer from comorbid rhinitis.

The prevalence of allergic rhinitis in the United States has been estimated to be between 15% and 40%, and this number is increasing.[14,15] There is a strong relationship between allergic rhinitis and asthma, and the two frequently coexist in the same patient. Patients with rhinitis have a 3 times higher risk of developing asthma than an individual without rhinitis, irrespective of the presence of atopy.[7,8] Asthma affects approximately 8% of the US population; however, the prevalence of asthma in patients with allergic rhinitis has been estimated to be as high as 40%. In contrast, up to 80% of asthmatic individuals also have allergic rhinitis.[16,17]

Allergic rhinitis tends to precede or occur at the same time as the development of asthma. In a study of 738 college students with 23 years of follow-up, the temporal relationship between rhinitis and asthma was assessed. Of those patients who had both allergic rhinitis and asthma, 44.8% developed nasal symptoms first and 20.7% developed upper and lower airway symptoms simultaneously. In patients with nonallergic rhinitis, 38.5% developed rhinitis first and 30.8% developed rhinitis and asthma at the same time.[7,18] In a retrospective review of 154 children with allergic rhinitis, approximately 20% of patients developed asthma within 10 years. Those with perennial allergic rhinitis were more likely to develop asthma than those with seasonal allergic rhinitis.[19] Linneberg and colleagues[20] examined the relationship between allergic rhinitis and asthma in 734 patients with confirmed IgE antibodies to pollen, animal dander, or dust mite. Over an 8-year follow-up period, the relative risk of developing asthma in patients with allergic rhinitis to pollen was 8.2, to animal dander was 18.9, and to dust mite was 46.5. At follow-up, 100% of patients with asthma also had allergic rhinitis.

Patients with both rhinitis and asthma tend to have more severe disease, which is more difficult and costly to control.[21–23] Large, population-based studies have demonstrated a link between the severity of both diseases. In a study of more than 25,000 asthmatic patients in the UK, those with concomitant allergic rhinitis experienced more doctor visits and were more often hospitalized for asthma. The presence of comorbid allergic rhinitis was associated with higher asthma-related drug costs.[24] In another study of almost 30,000 asthmatic patients in Japan, patients with concomitant allergic rhinitis were more likely to have uncontrolled asthma as defined by Global Initiative for Asthma guidelines than those without allergic rhinitis.[25] Conversely, Ponte and colleagues[26] demonstrated that poorly controlled asthma was associated with moderate to severe rhinitis.

Given the epidemiologic connection between allergic rhinitis and asthma, and the temporal relationship in which allergic rhinitis tends to precede the development of asthma, the Allergic Rhinitis and its Impact on Asthma guidelines have made several recommendations. Some recommendations were made in an attempt to prevent the development of both allergic rhinitis and asthma, including prophylactic avoidance of dust mite exposure and avoidance of occupational agent exposures, which contribute to the development atopic disease. In patients already sensitized to particular allergens, recommendations are made to avoid further exposure to indoor molds, animal dander, and occupational allergens.[27]

The link between the inflammatory response in the upper and lower airways is further substantiated by studies suggesting that the treatment of allergic rhinitis improves asthma outcomes. Optimal management of rhinitis may improve coexisting asthma. Several studies have shown a decrease in the frequency of asthma symptoms, improvement in lower airway function, and decrease in emergency room visits in patients using intranasal corticosteroids.[9–11,28–30] A recent metaanalysis conducted by Lohia and colleagues[31] examined the efficacy of intranasal corticosteroids on asthma outcomes. Data from 18 trials including a total of 2162 patients were analyzed. Nasal inhalation of corticosteroids resulted in improvement in asthma outcomes, including pulmonary function, bronchial reactivity, asthma symptom scores, asthma-specific quality of life, and rescue medication use. Crystal-Peters and colleagues[30] examined the rate of asthma-related emergency room visits and hospitalizations over a 1-year period. Of 4944 patients with allergic rhinitis and asthma, 3587 patients were treated for allergic rhinitis and 1357 were not. In the treated group, asthma-related hospitalizations decreased by 61%, and the incidence of 2 or more asthma-related emergency room visits decreased by 54% compared with the untreated group. These studies highlight the importance of recognizing the relationship between rhinitis and asthma, both in terms of reducing physical symptoms and in lowering health care costs.

Pathophysiologic Link

Both epidemiologic and pathophysiologic connections between rhinitis and asthma have been described. Several mechanisms have been proposed to explain the pathophysiologic link between the upper and lower airways. One proposed mechanism is that inflammatory products of the nose may be aspirated into the lower airways during an exacerbation of nasal inflammation. Although the aspiration of nasal contents may contribute to lower airway inflammation, there is significant evidence that a systemic response is involved. This mechanism is that of inflammatory cross-talk, in which local inflammation leads to upregulation of various inflammatory mediators, both locally and at distant sites within the respiratory tract. An additional proposed mechanism to explain the pathophysiologic link between the upper and lower airways is the neurogenic mechanism, in which neuronal stimulation in the nasal mucosa results in the release of neurotransmitters, which produce changes in the distal airway, including smooth muscle contraction.[32,33]

Several studies have demonstrated that allergic rhinitis and asthma are characterized by similar inflammatory processes, including the presence of similar proinflammatory mediators in response to the presence of an allergen. In previously sensitized individuals, the process is initiated when an antigen encounters high-affinity receptors on mast cell and basophil cell membranes. This reaction not only results in a local immune response, but also in a system-wide response, enabling the inflammatory reaction to reach other target organs through the circulatory system. During the early phase, an immediate hypersensitivity reaction occurs, during which preformed mediators are released from mast cells and basophils. This phase is characterized by rhinorrhea, sneezing, pruritus, cough, wheezing, and mucous production. In the late phase, which occurs 6 to 24 hours after initial exposure, eosinophils, basophils, and their progenitor cells are released from the bone marrow into the circulatory system.[3] Thus, allergic rhinitis is characterized not only by a local inflammatory response affecting the nasal airway, but also by a more diffuse involvement of the respiratory tract, even in the absence of clinical asthma.

In a study performed by Braunstahl and colleagues,[4] the upper and lower airways of 8 nonasthmatic patients with allergic rhinitis and 8 nonallergic healthy controls were evaluated after segmental bronchial provocation. The number of eosinophils and expression of interleukin (IL)-5 and eotaxin increased in both the nasal mucosa and blood of atopic individuals after segmental bronchial provocation; these changes were not observed in healthy controls. In a later study by the same group, segmental bronchial provocation was again undertaken to evaluate the role of mast cells and basophils in allergic inflammation of the upper and lower airway. Segmental bronchial provocation in nonasthmatic patients with allergic rhinitis resulted in a reduction in mast cells in the nasal mucosa owing to enhanced degranulation. There was a decrease in basophils in the bloodstream and an increase in basophils in the nasal and bronchial mucosa after segmental bronchial provocation in allergic patients that was not observed in nonallergic, healthy controls.[5] Conversely, nasal provocation was shown to result in the upregulation of adhesion molecules and eosinophils in both the upper and lower airway.[6]

Several studies also support the neurogenic mechanism for unified airway or united airway disease. Inflammation in the nose can lead to upregulation of neural activity, resulting in exaggerated responses, including sneezing, pruritus, and rhinorrhea, upon allergen exposure. Neural signals generated in the nose have been shown to affect distal respiratory sites.[34] In the presence of neuromediators, including substance P and calcitonin gene-related peptide, histamine and bradykinin are released, leading to increased vascular permeability and edema. Additionally, cholinergic neurotransmitters produce smooth muscle contraction, resulting in bronchoconstriction.[33]

RHINOSINUSITIS AND ASTHMA
Epidemiologic Relationship and Clinical Implications

Rhinosinusitis is defined as "a group of disorders characterized by inflammation of the mucosa of the nose and paranasal sinuses of at least 12 consecutive weeks."[35] Rhinosinusitis is associated with various symptoms including purulent rhinorrhea, nasal obstruction, facial pain or pressure, and decreased sense of smell. CRS affects 31 million patients in the United States each year, and the prevalence continues to grow. CRS represents a major health care issue, associated with frequent doctor visits, significant cost of medications for patients, and indirect costs incurred by the patient, including lost time from work or school.[36] According to the National Health and Nutrition Examination Survey, approximately 14% of Americans have CRS, and CRS accounts for 91.2 million health care visits per year.[37,38] A relationship between rhinosinusitis and asthma has been shown. The prevalence of asthma in the general population falls between 5% and 8%; however, the prevalence of asthma in patients with rhinosinusitis approaches 20%.[39–41] The Global Allergy and Asthma Network of Excellence conducted a large population-based, epidemiologic survey of more than 52,000 adults to determine the prevalence of asthma and rhinosinusitis in 12 European countries. There was a strong association between asthma and rhinosinusitis, with an odds ratio of 3.47 at all ages. The association was even stronger in those who reported allergic rhinitis in addition to CRS, with an odds ratio of 11.85.[41] Approximately 20% of patients with CRS have nasal polyps; in patients with chronic sinusitis with nasal polyps, the prevalence of asthma increases to 50%. This number is even higher in rhinosinusitis patients who ultimately undergo sinus surgery.[36,42,43]

The clinical association between sinusitis and asthma has been investigated. Multiple studies have demonstrated that the presence of comorbid CRS and asthma is associated with worse asthma outcomes. Using the results from the GA(2)LEN survey (Global Allergy and Asthma European Network), Elk and colleagues[44] studied the impact of CRS on pulmonary measures and quality-of-life outcomes in patients with asthma. Patients with both CRS and asthma had lower quality of life scores and poorer pulmonary function measures when compared with patients with asthma alone. In another study by ten Brinke and colleagues,[45] factors associated with frequent asthma exacerbation were investigated. In this study, severe sinonasal disease was associated with more frequent asthma exacerbations, with an odds ratio of 3.7.

The presence of asthma has been shown to be associated with worse sinus disease. In 1 study, patients with severe asthma were more likely to have severe sinonasal involvement, as measured by validated visual analog symptom scale and computed tomography (CT) scan, than those with mild to moderate asthma.[46] In another study of 89 patients with severe asthma, the degree of inflammation was assessed by CT score, pulmonary function testing, blood and sputum eosinophilia, and nitrous oxide in inhaled air. Significant associations were found between CT scan scores and peripheral blood eosinophil counts and exhaled nitric oxide levels. In this study, 84% of patients with severe asthma had an abnormal sinus CT scan.[47] A recent study of 187 patients with CRS aimed to determine whether the presence and severity of comorbid asthma impacts the clinical presentation of CRS. In this study, Lund-Mackay CT scores were significantly greater in patients with moderate or severe asthma compared with mild, intermittent, and nonasthmatic patients. The presence of allergic sensitization was highest in the moderate to severe asthma group, and the presence of nasal polyposis was significantly higher in the moderate to severe asthma group.[48]

The treatment of CRS has been shown to result in an improvement in asthma severity in those individuals with both diseases, although the evidence is inconsistent. Medical treatment of sinusitis alone has been shown in some studies to improve lower airway symptoms. Several studies have demonstrated that the use of intranasal corticosteroids results in decreased bronchial hyperresponsiveness. However, a recent multicenter, randomized, double-blind, placebo-controlled trial compared outcomes in patients treated with intranasal mometasone compared with placebo. There was no statistically significant difference in outcomes including asthma quality of life, lung function, or episodes of poorly controlled asthma in adults.[49]

Surgical treatment of CRS by endoscopic sinus surgery has been shown to improve both objective measures of pulmonary function and quality-of-life measures in patients with comorbid asthma. Several studies have shown decreased asthma medication use after sinus surgery. Additionally, continued medical therapy after sinus surgery has been shown to improve asthma control in long-term studies up to 6 years.[50–53]

Pathophysiologic Link

Rhinosinusitis and asthma seem to be 2 different manifestations of a similar pathophysiologic process in which eosinophils play a critical role. Whereas CRS represents a spectrum of disease with a variety of causative factors, eosinophil-mediated inflammation is common to most forms of rhinosinusitis, even in the absence of atopy.[36,39]

The mucosa of the respiratory tract, including the paranasal sinuses and bronchi, is composed of pseudostratified columnar epithelium. Chronic inflammation of the respiratory mucosa results in histologic changes, including basement membrane thickening, goblet cell hyperplasia, subepithelial edema, cellular infiltration, and mucous hypersecretion, which similarly affects the paranasal sinus and bronchial mucosa. In a histopathologic study performed by Dhong and colleagues,[54] the sinus mucosa of patients with and without asthma were examined. Basement membrane thickening, goblet cell hyperplasia, and eosinophil infiltration were found to be greater in the patients with sinusitis and comorbid asthma.

The inflammation of both CRS and asthma are characterized by similar inflammatory mediators and cells. Eosinophils and IL-5–producing lymphocytes are common to both disease processes. Key T-helper type 2–cell driven proinflammatory cytokines seen in both disease processes include IL-4, IL-5, and IL-13. IL-5 is responsible for promoting eosinophil production and preventing eosinophil apoptosis. Inflammatory mediators including regulated on activation normal T cell expressed and secreted (RANTES), eotaxin, and endothelial adhesion proteins are also seen in both CRS and asthma. RANTES and eotaxin facilitate transendothelial migration of eosinophils and movement of eosinophils into epithelium. Activation of adhesion proteins including intercellular adhesion molecule-1 and vascular cell adhesion molecule-1 leads to downstream effects, including transmigration of inflammatory cells. In the lower airway, this leads to airway narrowing and bronchospasm. With time, repeated insult results in permanent airway remodeling.[14]

The pathophysiologic similarities seen in CRS and asthma further support the unified airway or united airway disease model. The proposed mechanism of local and systemic inflammation via upregulation of inflammatory progenitors in the bone marrow provides a framework for the pathophysiologic similarities between CRS and asthma.

ASTHMA: EPIDEMIOLOGY AND CLINICAL PRESENTATION
Epidemiology

Asthma is a chronic lung disease characterized by bronchial hyperreactivity, resulting in episodic coughing, wheezing, chest tightness, and shortness of breath. More than 25 million children and adults suffer from asthma in the United States.[55,56] The number of people with asthma continues to increase. In 2001, 1 in 14 individuals, or 20 million people in the United States had asthma. By 2009, 1 in 12 people, or 25 million people had asthma. The overall prevalence of asthma in the United States is 7.8%. The prevalence of asthma is higher in children than in adults, with an estimated prevalence of 8.4%, making it the most common chronic disease of childhood.[13,57] Asthma is more likely to affect women and girls than men and boys. Increased asthma rates have disproportionately affected different ethnic groups. African American children are almost twice as likely to have asthma when compared with white children, with prevalence rates of 13.4% compared with 7.4%, respectively. African American children have experienced a disproportionately greater increase in asthma rates, an almost 50% increase between 2001 and 2009. Asthma also disproportionately affects people of different socioeconomic status, affecting 11.1% of those below the poverty level.[57] In addition to allergy, other risk factors for the development of asthma include environmental exposures, including tobacco smoke and pollution, respiratory infections, obesity, occupational exposures, and genetics.[13]

Morbidity and Mortality

Asthma is associated with significant morbidity and mortality in the United States. In 2010, the number of hospital outpatient department visits with asthma as the primary diagnosis was 1.3 million. The number of physician visits with asthma as the primary diagnosis in 2012 was 10.5 million. There were 1.6 million emergency department visits for asthma in 2013.[57] In 2015, there were a total of 3615 deaths attributable to asthma. Of that number, 219 deaths were in children and 3396 were in adults.

Asthma is not only a significant health issue, but also poses a major financial burden on society. With the increasing rates of asthma in the United States also comes increasing costs owing to medical costs, missed school or work days, hospitalizations, and early deaths. In the United States, the annual cost of asthma has increased by approximately 6% between 2002 and 2007, increasing from an estimated $53 million to $56 billion. Costs associated with asthma have a significant impact on both the national and individual levels. In 2015, the prevalence of asthma in those with private insurance was 7.0% compared with 13.6% in patients with Medicaid. Approximately 40% of uninsured and 11% of insured people with asthma are unable to afford their prescription medications.[57,58]

Clinical Presentation

Asthma is an inflammatory disorder characterized by symptoms including cough, wheezing, shortness of breath, or chest tightness. These symptoms are recurrent and are often associated with exposure to various triggers. Common triggers of asthma include inhalant allergen exposure, upper respiratory viral infection, and exposure to environmental irritants like smoke or pollution. Depending on the individual's trigger, symptoms may be worse at different times of the year or in different environments.[13]

The evaluation of a patient with asthma should include a thorough history, including history of atopic disease. Patients should be questioned about the presence of both upper and lower respiratory symptoms. Nasal symptoms including nasal congestion, rhinorrhea, hyposmia, anosmia, postnasal drip, and sneezing should be elicited. Patients should be asked about triggers of their symptoms, whether symptoms are worse in a particular location or more severe during a particular season. Because asthma is, in part, a heritable disease, it is important to gather a thorough family history of asthma and/or allergy. The diagnosis and management of asthma is discussed in detail (See John H. Krouse's article, "Asthma Management for the Otolaryngologist," in this issue for further details).

ALLERGIC RHINITIS AND OTHER COMORBIDITIES
Laryngitis

Although there has been extensive research over the past 2 decades aiming to characterize the relationship of the upper and lower airways, much of the work has focused on allergic rhinitis, sinusitis, and asthma. The role of the larynx in the unified airway is less well understood. Although there has been anecdotal evidence of the connection between allergy and vocal dysfunction, there are few controlled studies examining this.[59] The larynx is positioned between the upper and lower airways, and therefore may be considered a part of the unified airway. In acute laryngitis, diffuse inflammation involving the supraglottis, glottis, and subglottis can be seen. In contrast, chronic laryngitis is characterized by inflammatory changes primarily at the level of the vocal folds. Several studies have examined the role of allergy in both acute and chronic laryngitis. Corey and colleagues[60] described and differentiated between the 2 forms of laryngitis. In acute allergic laryngitis, upon exposure to an allergen, there is rapid edema of the lips, tongue, pharynx, and larynx. This potentially life-threatening response may be associated with cutaneous symptoms, dyspnea, and tachycardia. Chronic laryngitis has a significantly less aggressive presentation. These patients typically have mild vocal fold edema and thick mucous of the glottis and supraglottis. Chronic laryngeal inflammation can result in dysphonia, throat clearing, and cough.

Several studies have attempted to define the mechanism by which allergic laryngitis occurs.[61,62] Two underlying processes have been proposed to result in allergic laryngitis. The first proposed mechanism suggests that impaired nasal breathing results in altered resonance characteristics of the upper airway, resulting in dysphonia in the allergic patient.[63] The second, more recently proposed mechanism, suggests that postnasal drip leads to laryngeal irritation and subsequent harmful behaviors including coughing and throat clearing.[62,64] Dworkin and Stachler[62] proposed a model for laryngitis resulting from inhalant allergen exposure, describing 3 contributory mechanisms. First, local inflammation in the nose or sinuses produces a system-wide inflammatory response by upregulation of inflammatory mediators in the circulatory system and by local increase mucous production. Second, increased mucous produced in the upper airways is transported to the pharynx and ultimately to the larynx. Last, this mucous acts as an irritant on the pharynx and larynx, resulting in compensatory behaviors, including throat clearing and coughing. These behaviors result in histologic changes to the laryngeal mucosa.[62,65] Finally, some suggest that allergic laryngitis results from the systemic propagation of local inflammation to involve the entire respiratory tract, that is, the unified airway.[59]

Epidemiology and Clinical Implications

The association between allergic rhinitis and laryngitis has been shown in multiple studies. Simberg and colleagues[66] performed a survey in 49 allergic patients and 54 nonallergic controls in which the frequency of various vocal complaints was assessed. Patients in the allergy group had significantly more severe voice symptoms than nonallergic controls. These differences remained when controlling for asthma. In another study conducted by Millqvist and colleagues,[67] 30 patients with confirmed allergy and 30 nonallergic controls were evaluated for subjective voice dysfunction using the Voice Handicap Index, a validated questionnaire for the evaluation of voice quality. During allergy season, patients with allergy reported significantly more respiratory and voice symptoms than did controls.

The relationship was investigated further in direct provocation studies.[68,69] Reidy and colleagues[68] developed transoral provocation using nebulized antigen. Dworkin and colleagues[69] found that when using a high concentration of antigen, patients developed vocal fold edema and erythema, increased secretions, coughing, hoarseness, and respiratory issues. These reactions lead to early termination of the study owing to safety concerns. In an attempt to control for potential confounders, including pulmonary reactions, Roth and colleagues[70] conducted a similar study using transoral provocation, but excluded those patients with airway reactivity on methacholine challenge. In this double-blind, placebo-controlled study, the effect of antigen challenge on subglottic pressure was compared with the effect from saline placebo. All patients had significant increase in subglottic pressure after antigen presentation.

The relationship between allergy and vocal dysfunction has been shown; however, further investigations must be undertaken to determine the mechanism behind allergic laryngitis. Patients with dysphonia or cough should be evaluated for comorbidities including allergic rhinitis, sinusitis, and asthma.

Conjunctivitis

Conjunctivitis is an inflammation of the conjunctiva caused by a variety of agents, including allergens. Ocular allergy represents a heterogeneous group of disorders with different pathophysiologic mechanisms, physical manifestations, and treatment responses, and incudes acute allergic conjunctivitis, allergic conjunctivitis, vernal keratoconjunctivitis, and atopic conjunctivitis, among others. Allergic conjunctivitis is an inflammatory response of the conjunctiva to environmental allergen and often occurs in conjunction with allergic rhinitis.[71] Signs and symptoms of conjunctivitis include conjunctival hyperemia, chemosis, itching, tearing, and/or mucoid discharge. These signs and symptoms are the result of an immune response triggered in a previously sensitized individual. Upon subsequent exposure of an individual's ocular surface to a particular allergen, allergen-specific IgE receptors on conjunctival mast cells are activated, resulting in mast cell degranulation. Inflammatory mediators, including histamine, prostaglandins, and leukotrienes, contribute to the manifestations of ocular allergy.[72] Allergic conjunctivitis of this type affects the tarsal conjunctiva and eyelid but spares the cornea.[71]

Epidemiology and Clinical Implications

Allergic conjunctivitis is common, affecting up to 40% of the population in the United States.[73] Between 40% and 60% of patients with atopy are affected by ocular symptoms.[73,74] Using data from the third National Health and Nutrition Examination Survey, the prevalence of allergic conjunctivitis has been estimated. Of the 20,010 individuals surveyed, 6.4% of the population reported ocular symptoms alone, 16.5% reported nasal symptoms alone, 29.7% reported both nasal and ocular symptoms, and 47.4% were asymptomatic. In this study, 40% of surveyed individuals reported at least 1 occurrence of ocular symptoms in their lifetime. Ocular symptoms tend to be present throughout all decades of life, in contrast with isolated nasal symptoms or combined nasal and ocular symptoms.[73] There is a strong epidemiologic connection between allergic conjunctivitis and allergic rhinitis. The epidemiologic link between allergic conjunctivitis and rhinitis is so strong that epidemiologic studies rarely separate the clinical entities; rather, allergic rhinoconjunctivitis has been studied more thoroughly. The connection between allergic rhinitis and allergic conjunctivitis is further substantiated by studies showing that treatment of allergic rhinitis with intranasal steroids improves ocular symptoms as well.[75]

SUMMARY

The upper and lower airways are connected both epidemiologically and pathophysiologically. Local and systemic inflammatory responses to allergen exposure have given rise to notion of the unified airway or united airway disease. Otolaryngologists encounter patients with upper airway symptoms, including nasal obstruction, nasal congestion, rhinorrhea, and sneezing in daily practice. Therefore, the otolaryngologist should familiarize himself or herself with the signs and symptoms of lower airway disease which often accompany upper airway pathology. Although the diagnosis and management pf asthma is not traditionally thought to fall within the purview of an otolaryngology practice, the otolaryngologist may be the first to suspect lower airway pathology in a patient presenting with upper airway complaints. In light of the evidence that treatment of lower airway disease impacts therapeutic outcomes in upper airway disease, and vice versa, the importance of expedient diagnosis and management of asthma is clear.

REFERENCES

1. Pillsbury HC 3rd, Krouse JH, Marple BF, et al. The impact/role of asthma in otolaryngology. Otolaryngol Head Neck Surg 2007;136:157.
2. Passalacqua G, Ciprandi G, Canonica GW. United airways disease: therapeutic aspects. Thorax 2000;55(Suppl 2):S26–7.
3. Giavina-Bianchi P, Aun MV, Takejima P, et al. United airway disease: current perspectives. J Asthma Allergy 2016;9:93–100.
4. Braunstahl GJ, Kleinjan A, Overbeek SE, et al. Segmental bronchial provocation induces nasal inflammation in allergic rhinitis patients. Am J Respir Crit Care Med 2000;161:2051–7.
5. Braunstahl GJ, Overbeek SE, Fokkens WJ, et al. Segmental bronchoprovocation in allergic rhinitis patients affects mast cell and basophil numbers in nasal and bronchial mucosa. Am J Respir Crit Care Med 2001;164:858–65.

6. Braunstahl GJ, Overbeek SE, Kleinjan A, et al. Nasal allergen provocation induces adhesion molecule expression and tissue eosinophilia in upper and lower airways. J Allergy Clin Immunol 2001;107:469–76.

7. Settipane RJ, Hagy GW, Settipane GA. Long-term risk factors for developing asthma and allergic rhinitis: a 23-year follow-up study of college students. Allergy Proc 1994;15:21–5.

8. Guerra S, Sherrill DL, Martinez FD, et al. Rhinitis as an independent risk factor for adult-onset asthma. J Allergy Clin Immunol 2002;109:419–25.

9. Stelmach R, do Patrocínio T Nunes M, Ribeiro M, et al. Effect of treating allergic rhinitis with corticosteroids in patients with mild-to-moderate persistent asthma. Chest 2005;128:3140–7.

10. Watson WT, Becker AB, Simons FE. Treatment of allergic rhinitis with intranasal corticosteroids in patients with mild asthma: effect on lower airway responsiveness. J Allergy Clin Immunol 1993;91:97–101.

11. Fuhlbrigge AL, Adams RJ. The effect of treatment of allergic rhinitis on asthma morbidity, including emergency department visits. Curr Opin Allergy Clin Immunol 2003;3:29–32.

12. Bousquet J, Van Cauwenberge P, Khalaev N, ARIA Workshop Group, World Health Organization. Allergic rhinitis and its impact on asthma. J Allergy Clin Immunol 2001;108(5):147–336.

13. Toskala E, Kennedy DW. Asthma risk factors. Int Forum Allergy Rhinol 2015; 5(Suppl 1):S11–6.

14. Krouse JH, Brown RW, Fineman SM, et al. Asthma and the unified airway. Otolaryngol Head Neck Surg 2007;136:S75–106.

15. Meltzer EO. The relationships of rhinitis and asthma. Allergy Asthma Proc 2005; 26:336–40.

16. Corren J. Allergic rhinitis and asthma: how important is the link? J Allergy Clin Immunol 1997;99:S781–6.

17. Custovic A, Simpson A. The role of inhalant allergens in allergic airways disease. J Investig Allergol Clin Immunol 2012;22(6):393–401.

18. Greisner WA 3rd, Settipane RJ, Settipane GA. Co-existence of asthma and allergic rhinitis: a 23-year follow-up study of college students. Allergy Asthma Proc 1998;19:185–8.

19. Linna O, Kokkonen J, Lukin M. A 10-year prognosis for childhood allergic rhinitis. Acta Paediatr 1992;81:100–2.

20. Linneberg A, Henrik Nielsen N, Frølund L, et al. The link between allergic rhinitis and allergic asthma: a prospective population-based study. The Copenhagen Allergy Study. Allergy 2002;57:1048–52.

21. Antonicelli L, Micucci C, Voltolini S, et al. Relationship between ARIA classification and drug treatment in allergic rhinitis and asthma. Allergy 2007;62:1064–70.

22. Halpern MT, Schmier JK, Richner R, et al. Allergic rhinitis: a potential cause of increased asthma medication use, costs, and morbidity. J Asthma 2004;41: 117–26.

23. Greisner WA 3rd, Settipane RJ, Settipane GA. The course of asthma parallels that of allergic rhinitis: a 23 year follow-up study of college students. Allergy Asthma Proc 2000;21(6):371–5.

24. Price D, Zhang Q, Kocevar VS, et al. Effect of a concomitant diagnosis of allergic rhinitis on asthma-related health care use by adults. Clin Exp Allergy 2005;35: 282–7.

25. Ohta K, Bousquet PJ, Aizawa H, et al. Prevalence and impact of rhinitis in asthma. SACRA, a cross-sectional nation-wide study in Japan. Allergy 2011;66: 1287–95.

26. Ponte EV, Franco R, Nascimento HF, et al. Lack of control of severe asthma is associated with co-existence of moderate-to-severe rhinitis. Allergy 2008;63: 564–9.

27. Brozek JL, Bousquet J, Baena-Cagnani CE, et al. Allergic rhinitis and its impact on asthma (ARIA) guidelines: 2010 revision. J Allergy Clin Immunol 2010;126: 466–76.

28. Pedersen B, Dahl R, Lindqvist N, et al. Nasal inhalation of the glucocorticoid budesonide from a spacer for the treatment of patients with pollen rhinitis and asthma. Allergy 1990;45:451–6.

29. Foresi A, Pelucchi A, Gherson G, et al. Once daily intranasal fluticasone propionate (200 micrograms) reduces nasal symptoms and inflammation but also attenuates the increase in bronchial responsiveness during the pollen season in allergic rhinitis. J Allergy Clin Immunol 1996;98:274–82.

30. Crystal-Peters J, Neslusan C, Crown WH, et al. Treating allergic rhinitis in patients with comorbid asthma: the risk of asthma-related hospitalizations and emergency department visits. J Allergy Clin Immunol 2002;109:57–62.

31. Lohia S, Schlosser RJ, Soler ZM. Impact of intranasal corticosteroids on asthma outcomes in allergic rhinitis: a meta-analysis. Allergy 2013;68:569–79.

32. Feng CH, Miller MD, Simon RA. The united allergic airway: connections between allergic rhinitis, asthma, and chronic sinusitis. Am J Rhinol Allergy 2012;26: 187–90.

33. Georgopoulos R, Krouse JH, Toskala E. Why otolaryngologists and asthma are a good match: the allergic rhinitis-asthma connection. Otolaryngol Clin North Am 2014;47:1–12.

34. Sarin S, Undem B, Sanico A, et al. The role of the nervous system in rhinitis. J Allergy Clin Immunol 2006;118(5):999–1016.

35. Benninger MS, Ferguson BJ, Hadley JA, et al. Adult chronic rhinosinusitis: definitions, diagnosis, epidemiology and pathophysiology. Otolaryngol Head Neck Surg 2003;129(3 Suppl):S1–32.

36. Meltzer EO, Hamilos DL, Hadley JA, et al. Rhinosinusitis: establishing definitions for clinical research and patient care. Otolaryngol Head Neck Surg 2004;131: S1–62.

37. Adams PF, Hendershot GE, Marano MA. Current estimates from the National Health Interview Survey, 1996. Vital Health Stat 10 1999;(200):1–203.

38. Smith WM, Davidson TM, Murphy C. Regional variations in chronic rhinosinusitis, 2003-2006. Otolaryngol Head Neck Surg 2009;141:347–52.

39. Jani A, Hamilos D. Current thinking on the relationship between rhinosinusitis and asthma. J Asthma 2005;42:1–7.

40. Bachert C, Vignola M, Gevaert P, et al. Allergic rhinitis, rhinosinusitis, and asthma: one airway disease. Immunol Allergy Clin N Am 2004;24:19–43.

41. Jarvis D, Newson R, Lotvall J, et al. Asthma in adults and its association with chronic rhinosinusitis: the GA2LEN survey in Europe. Allergy 2012;67:91–8.

42. Hamilos DL. Chronic sinusitis. J Allergy Clin Immunol 2000;106:213–27.

43. Senior BA, Kennedy DW, Tanabodee J, et al. Long-term impact of functional endoscopic sinus surgery on asthma. Otolaryngol Head Neck Surg 1999;121: 66–8.

44. Elk A, Middelveld RJ, Bertilsson H, et al. Chronic rhinosinusitis in asthma is a negative predictor of quality of life: results from the Swedish GA(2)LEN survey. Allergy 2013;68:1314–21.
45. ten Brinke A, Sterk PJ, Masclee AA, et al. Risk factors of frequent exacerbations in difficult-to-treat asthma. Eur Respir J 2005;26:812–8.
46. Bresciani M, Paradis L, Des Roches A, et al. Rhinosinusitis in severe asthma. J Allergy Clin Immunol 2001;107:73–80.
47. ten Brinke A, Grootendorst DC, Schmidt JT, et al. Chronic sinusitis in severe asthma is related to sputum eosinophilia. J Allergy Clin Immunol 2002;109:621–6.
48. Lin DC, Chandra RK, Tan BK, et al. Association between severity of asthma and degree of chronic rhinosinusitis. Am J Rhinol Allergy 2011;25:205–8.
49. American Lung Association–Asthma Clinical Research Centers' Writing Committee, Dixon AE, Castro M, Cohen RI, et al. Efficacy of nasal mometasone for the treatment of chronic sinonasal disease in patients with inadequately controlled asthma. J Allergy Clin Immunol 2015;135:701–9.e5.
50. Batra PS, Kern RC, Tripathi A, et al. Outcome analysis of endoscopic sinus surgery in patients with nasal polyps and asthma. Laryngoscope 2003;113:1703–6.
51. Slavin RG. Asthma and sinusitis. J Allergy Clin Immunol 1992;90:534–7.
52. Jankowski R, Moneret-Vautrin DA, Goets R, et al. Incidence of medico-surgical treatment for nasal polyps on the development of associated asthma. Rhinology 1992;30:249–58.
53. Alobid I, Benítez P, Bernal-Sprekelsen M, et al. The impact of asthma and aspirin sensitivity on quality of life of patients with nasal polyposis. Qual Life Res 2005;14:789–93.
54. Dhong HJ, Kim HY, Cho DY. Histopathologic characteristics of chronic sinusitis with bronchial asthma. Acta Otolaryngol 2005;125:169–76.
55. American Lung Association. Asthma & children fact sheet. 2014. Available at: http://www.lung.org/lung-disease/asthma/resources/facts-and-figures/asthma-children-fact-sheet.html. Accessed May 14, 2015.
56. American Lung Association. Asthma in adults fact sheet. 2012. Available at: http://www.lung.org/lungdisease/asthma/resources/facts-and-figures/asthmain-adults.html. Accessed May 14, 2015.
57. Center for Disease Control and Prevention. Asthma: data, statistics, and surveillance. 2016. Available at: https://www.cdc.gov/asthma/asthmadata.htm. Accessed May 6, 2017.
58. American College of Allergy, Asthma & Immunology Allergy. Asthma information. 2014. Available at: http://acaai.org/asthma/about. Accessed April 16, 2017.
59. Roth DF, Ferguson BJ. Vocal allergy: recent advances in understanding the role of allergy in dysphonia. Curr Opin Otolaryngol Head Neck Surg 2010;18:176–81.
60. Corey JP, Gungor A, Karnell M. Allergy for the laryngologist. Otolaryngol Clin North Am 1998;31:189–205.
61. Cohn JR, Sataloff RT, Branton C. Response of asthma-related voice dysfunction to allergen immunotherapy: a case report of confirmation by methacholine challenge. J Voice 2001;15:558–60.
62. Dworkin JP, Stachler RJ. Management of the patient with laryngitis. In: Krouse JH, Derebery MJ, Chadwick SJ, editors. Managing the allergic patient. Philadelphia: Elsevier; 2007. p. 233–72.
63. Brodnitz FS. Allergy of the larynx. Otolaryngol Clin North Am 1971;4:579–82.
64. Chadwick SJ. Allergy and the contemporary laryngologist. Otolaryngol Clin North Am 2003;36:957–88.

65. Krouse JH, Altman KW. Rhinogenic laryngitis, cough, and the unified airway. Otolaryngol Clin North Am 2010;43:111–21.

66. Simberg S, Sala E, Tuomainen J, et al. Vocal symptoms and allergy-a pilot study. J Voice 2009;23:136–9.

67. Millqvist E, Bende M, Brynnel M, et al. Voice change in seasonal allergic rhinitis. J Voice 2008;22:512–5.

68. Reidy PM, Dworkin JP, Krouse JH. Laryngeal effects of antigen stimulation challenge with perennial allergen Dermatophagoides pteronyssinus. Otolaryngol Head Neck Surg 2003;128(4):301–7.

69. Dworkin JP, Reidy PM, Stachler RJ, et al. Effects of sequential Dermatophagoides pteronyssinus antigen stimulation on anatomy and physiology of the larynx. Ear Nose Throat J 2009;88:793–9.

70. Roth DF, Verdolini K, Carroll T, et al. Laryngeal allergy, nothing to sniff at: evidence for laryngeal allergy. American Academy of Otolaryngologic Allergy 68th Annual Meeting. San Diego, CA, October 2, 2009.

71. Bousquet J, Khaltaev N, Cruz AA, et al. Allergic rhinitis and its impact on asthma (ARIA) 2008 update (in collaboration with the World Health Organization, GA(2) LEN and AllerGen). Allergy 2008;63(Suppl 86):8–160.

72. Bielory BP, O'Brien TP, Bielory L. Management of seasonal allergic conjunctivitis: guide to therapy. Acta Ophthalmol 2012;90:399–407.

73. Singh K, Axelrod S, Bielory L. The epidemiology of ocular and nasal allergy in the United States, 1988-1994. J Allergy Clin Immunol 2010;126:778–83.

74. Leonardi A, Bogacka E, Fauquert JL, et al. Ocular allergy: recognizing and diagnosing hypersensitivity disorders of the ocular surface. Allergy 2012;67:1327–37.

75. Bielory L, Chun Y, Bielory BP, et al. Impact of mometasone furoate nasal spray on individual ocular symptoms of allergic rhinitis: a meta-analysis. Allergy 2011;66: 686–93.

Asthma Management for the Otolaryngologist

John H. Krouse, MD, PhD, MBA

KEYWORDS

• Asthma • Cough • Pulmonary function testing • Unified airway

KEY POINTS

- Asthma is an reversible, obstructive, inflammatory disease of the lower airways that is characterized by cough, wheezing, and shortness of breath.
- Patients with asthma may present with cough alone, often occurring at night.
- Patients presenting with nighttime cough should always have asthma considered as part of the differential diagnosis.
- Owing to system-wide inflammatory effects, otolaryngologists should consider the potential presence of asthma in all patients presenting with allergic rhinitis or chronic rhinosinusitis.
- Asthma can be classified on the basis of severity and chronicity of symptoms, and treated to optimize the patient's level of symptom control.

INTRODUCTION

Asthma is a common inflammatory condition of the lower respiratory system.[1] It is found in all age groups, from infants to older adults, and presents a major disease burden that affects approximately 300 million persons worldwide.[2] Patients with asthma report a cluster of 3 primary symptoms, including cough, wheezing, and shortness of breath (dyspnea). For many patients, their only symptoms may be a dry cough, often occurring at night, and frequently severe enough to wake them from sleep. Because these symptoms overlap with other common conditions, the diagnosis of asthma is sometimes elusive, and patients with asthma often are misclassified, with unsuccessful treatment and no resolution of their symptoms.

Asthma is a type of obstructive lung disease. With obstruction, patients are able to inspire at relatively normal levels, but have difficulty exhaling fully owing to both narrowing of the lower airways and loss of elasticity of the bronchioles. As a result, air becomes trapped in the lungs, which limits the amount of air exchange and can ultimately decrease oxygenation. In asthma, as opposed to chronic obstructive

Disclosures: None.

School of Medicine, University of Texas Rio Grande Valley, 1201 West, University Drive, Edinburg, Texas 78539, USA

E-mail address: john.krouse@utrgv.edu

Otolaryngol Clin N Am 50 (2017) 1065–1076
http://dx.doi.org/10.1016/j.otc.2017.08.006

oto.theclinics.com

pulmonary disease, the airway obstruction is at least partially reversible, and the use of a bronchodilating agent such as albuterol will improve expiration and relieve symptoms.

It is important for otolaryngologists to recognize that asthma represents only 1 focused aspect of a broader spectrum of inflammatory respiratory symptoms and that many patients seeking care for conditions such as allergic rhinitis and chronic rhinosinusitis also have concurrent asthma. The concept of the "unified airway" has become well-accepted over the past several decades, and has allowed otolaryngologists to better understand and appreciate the comorbidity of upper and lower airway inflammation among patients with common sinonasal complaints.[3] Recognition of these inflammatory comorbidities prompted the World Health Organization in 2002 to state: "When considering a diagnosis of rhinitis or asthma, an evaluation of both the upper and lower airways should be made."[4]

This article focuses on the management of asthma for otolaryngologists. Because otolaryngologists commonly encounter patients with unified airway diseases such as asthma, many of whom may have undiagnosed disease, it is important for these physicians to recognize the symptoms of asthma, understand the basic elements of diagnosis, and appreciate common approaches to the management of symptoms and control of the underlying disease in these patients.

PATHOPHYSIOLOGY OF ASTHMA

The pathophysiology of asthma involves a variety of complex and interactive processes that result in acute and chronic airway inflammation. The majority of patients with asthma have inflammation that is primarily driven by T-helper 2 cells, with activation of cellular and humoral mediators including mast cells, eosinophils and lymphocytes, as well as numerous interleukins (IL-4, IL-5, and IL-13), chemokines, and other cytokines.[1,5] In many individuals, this process begins in early childhood, resulting in chronic and progressive inflammatory changes in the lower airway. In others, asthma presents in adults, with little prior history of inflammatory or atopic disease in childhood.

Tissue changes occur in patients with asthma, and are generally progressive with time. Much of this inflammation can be subacute, but with exposure to various triggering stimuli can be unmasked, allowing the acute expression of symptoms among affected patients.[6] A variety of intrinsic and extrinsic factors can be involved in both the pathogenesis and expression of asthma, including underlying atopy, sensitization, and exposure to allergic antigens, exposure to tobacco smoke, infectious exacerbations, and contact with nonspecific irritants. These inflammatory influences provoke characteristic changes in the respiratory tract, including epithelial shedding, goblet cell hyperplasia, hypertrophy of submucosal mucus glands, subepithelial fibrosis with collagen deposition, smooth muscle hypertrophy, and vascular leakage. These changes are expressed through the cardinal symptoms of cough, wheezing, and dyspnea.[7]

The changes in the lungs that occur over time worsen as the disease progresses, and although initially they can be reversed with treatment, they will become irreversible with chronicity. These changes are described broadly as "remodeling," representing structural changes in the bronchioles that cause decrease function and increased patient symptoms. These pathophysiologic changes can be described in 3 phases: acute inflammatory, chronic inflammatory, and irreversible (remodeling).

Acute inflammatory changes
- Epithelial cell edema
- Muscle constriction

- Vascular leakage
- Mucus hypersecretion

Chronic inflammatory changes

- Loss of epithelial cells
- Exposure of nerve endings
- Loss of cilia
- Increased goblet cells
- Submucosal fibrosis
- Increased muscle mass

Irreversible (remodeling) changes

- Dense deposition of collagen
- Marked increase in muscle mass
- Loss of epithelial cells
- Loss of elasticity

As these progressive changes occur, there is narrowing of the lumen of the airway, which causes increased wheezing, decreased airway diameter for respiration, and increased frequency of mucus plugging and airway obstruction. Because of these changes, air trapping in the lungs becomes common and the patient experiences increasing difficulty in expiration. It is these contributors to airway narrowing that are primary drivers to the symptoms that patients experience during asthmatic episodes and exacerbations.[8]

PRESENTATION

Although many patients will seek treatment for asthma when they are experiencing wheezing or shortness of breath (dyspnea), there are a number of individuals with chronic cough who may have asthma that has not been recognized or diagnosed. Many patients with asthma only recognize acute exacerbations as characterizing an episode of asthma, yet ignore the mild wheezing and nighttime cough that become accepted as normal. It is important for otolaryngologists to consider asthma among all patients presenting to their offices with cough, especially nighttime cough that awakens them from sleep.

Asthma symptoms may be present persistently, but are often episodic. They can occur throughout the year or may have a predilection to occur seasonally. Asthma symptoms may be exacerbated with a concurrent viral upper or lower respiratory infection, and can be worse with exposure to both allergens and nonallergic triggers. Cough again may be the sole symptom of asthma in some patients, so a careful differential and diagnostic approach must be used by treating otolaryngologists to accurately assess this symptom and its causes.

DIAGNOSIS

As with most inflammatory diseases, a careful history is important in assisting with the diagnostic process. Patients with asthma often have a family history of asthma or atopic disease, because there is some genetic predisposition to the development of asthma. Adult patients may have experienced asthma in childhood, only to outgrow its symptoms before the development of adult disease. In addition, many patients with asthma will have a prior history of allergic rhinitis or allergic eczema, with asthma symptoms presenting only later in childhood or in adulthood. In fact, the presence of allergic rhinitis seems to predispose individuals to the development of asthma later in life.[9]

Patients with asthma will often present with cough, which is usually described as dry and nonproductive. It can occur throughout the day, but a nighttime cough is frequently characteristic of asthma. The presence of cough is nonspecific, and should prompt the otolaryngologist to consider not only a diagnosis of asthma, but other triggering conditions such as laryngopharyngeal reflux disease. A more specific but less common symptom at presentation is that of wheezing, which is representative of worsening bronchospasm among patients with asthma. As the disease worsens, patients will complain of difficult breathing and chest tightness, both of which are symptoms of more severe asthma.

The history should also include an assessment of any triggers or antecedent events that may have caused the symptoms to occur. These should include both allergic and nonallergic triggers, as well as a prior history of allergic or atopic diseases. In addition, inquiry should be made about prior treatments, both medical and adjuvant, that might have been used to alleviate the patient's symptoms.

The physical examination in a patient with asthma may be essentially normal, even in patients with more severe disease. Because of the variability in symptom expression, patients may be relatively free of findings at an office visit. Common signs that may be present include a dry cough, end-expiratory wheezes on chest auscultation, or even chest retractions with severe exacerbation. In patients having respiratory distress owing to asthma, patients will display accessory muscle use for breathing, tachypnea, and even cyanosis. Patients expressing these severe signs will need emergency treatment in a critical care setting.

The primary diagnostic procedure that is used for the assessment of patients with asthma is pulmonary function testing. Although many pulmonary function test measures exist, the most appropriate and useful in assessment of asthma is spirometry, with measurements made both before and after the use of a short-acting β-2 agonist as a bronchodilator. In spirometry, the patient is asked to take a full inhalation and then to maximally and rapidly exhale into a measurement device. Three measurements are generally recorded. The patient then inhales the short-acting bronchodilator, and after 10 minutes repeats the test.

The major indices that are used to assess airflow during spirometry are:

- Forced expiratory volume in 1 second (FEV_1), and
- Forced vital capacity (FVC).

These findings are compared with benchmarks that are normalized for the specific demographic reference group for the patient and then assessed. In patients with obstructive lung diseases such as asthma, the FEV_1 is reduced, generally to less than 80% of the predicted value, the FVC is maintained near normal levels, and the FEV_1/FVC ratio is reduced. In patients with asthma, which is a reversible obstructive airway disease, the FEV_1 will improve after the administration of a β-2 agonist, with an improvement of 12% or more generally considered diagnostic of asthma among patients with obstruction.

In some patients who have subclinical or intermittent asthma, pulmonary function testing may be nondiagnostic when performed as described. In those patients, it can be useful to challenge their airways to see if they will respond to inhalation of a triggering agent. This procedure can help to assess the presence of airway inflammation that may be otherwise missed. In bronchial provocation, an agent such as methacholine or histamine can be administered by inhalational challenge to see if testing can elicit a decline in FEV_1. In patients with subclinical inflammation, a decrease in FEV_1 of 20% or more with progressive challenge indicates the presence of asthma and can be diagnostic in the absence of routine testing.

Other indicators that can be measured during spirometry are the peak expiratory flow rate and forced expiratory flow rate between the 25% percentile and the 75% percentile of the FVC. The peak expiratory flow rate is more of an expression of airflow in the large airways, and may underrepresent the importance of disease in the small airways most affected by asthma. It is therefore a late indicator of change. In contrast, the forced expiratory flow rate between the 25% percentile and the 75% percentile of the FVC is an assessment of very small airways, and may be overly sensitive to change, making it a less useful clinical indicator than the FEV_1.

Other tests can be useful in the diagnosis of asthma, but are used less frequently. One of the more common measures is exhaled nitric oxide testing, which assesses the presence of nitric oxide as a proxy for airway inflammation, and can be useful in both diagnosing the presence of asthma and in assessing the response to treatment. In some patients, chest radiographs can be useful, as can serum measurements of specific or total immunoglobulin E. Skin testing for inhalant allergy can also be useful in assessing the presence of allergic triggers that may be important in symptom expression and exacerbation.

CONTROL

The ultimate goal for the management of the patient with asthma is the establishment of control. Because asthma is a chronic inflammatory disease, current therapeutic methods do not consider the objective of management to be the establishment of cure, but rather the ability to provide the patient with freedom for symptoms and a normal quality of life. Although theoretically the goal of therapy would be to eliminate all underlying inflammation and to prevent the progression of disease, the facility of current diagnostic testing does not permit a sufficiently adequate assessment to allow this evaluation.

Two concepts are important in facilitating the management of patients with asthma: severity and control. Severity is the intrinsic intensity of the disease process, which allows both initial establishment of therapy and the adjustment of therapy over time. Control is the degree to which the manifestations of asthma, such as symptoms, functional impairments, and risks of untoward events, are minimized and optimal patient quality of life is achieved.[1] The goal of therapy can be seen to maintain complete control of symptoms over time with the lowest dose of medications necessary and with the fewest side effects. Specifically, these goals are to:

- Gain and maintain control of asthma symptoms;
- Maintain normal activity levels, including exercise;
- Prevent asthma exacerbations;
- Avoid adverse effects from asthma medications; and
- Prevent asthma mortality.[10]

Levels of asthma control are generally assessed using a variety of clinical indicators, including:

- Daytime symptoms;
- Limitations of activities;
- Nocturnal symptoms/awakenings;
- Need for reliever or rescue treatment; and
- Exacerbations.[10]

When asthma is under complete control, the patient should be experiencing none of these clinical findings. They should be free of all symptoms, day and night, and not need to use any medications for acute relief of symptoms. Asthma can be considered partially controlled with the patient experiencing some of these clinical findings, but when patients are frequently symptomatic and require frequent medication use for acute symptom treatment, their asthma would be considered uncontrolled.

Although patients may be assessed clinically by simply inquiring about each of the specific indicators noted, there are validated measures of asthma control that can be used for both clinical and research indications. Two of these measures include the Asthma Control Test (available: http://www.asthmacontrol.com) and the Asthma Control Questionnaire (available: http://www.qoltech.co.uk/acq.html).

MANAGEMENT

Because the current strategic initiative is to assist the patient to achieve asthma control, the goal is to use patient-based indicators of function to guide therapy as opposed to relying on assessment of pulmonary function by spirometry. Control is a dynamic indicator and reflects the patient's level of function better than a static assessment of severity of lung function impairment alone. The establishment and maintenance of control requires an active partnership between the patient, the patient's family, and the physician, and involves the use of both educational interventions and appropriate medications to achieve success.

Because asthma exacerbations can be triggered by environmental exposures to both allergic and nonallergic factors, understanding these triggers and avoiding them as possible is an important strategy. Although it would seem to be wise to avoid allergenic exposures, there is no compelling evidence that avoidance strategies are effective in reducing the clinical burden of disease. In contrast, the avoidance of tobacco exposure does decrease symptomatic expression and improve control among patients with asthma.

There is also evidence that treating allergic rhinitis with medications and immunotherapy can be beneficial in reducing asthma symptoms and improving control.[11] Although the benefits reported vary in different trials, both antihistamines and intranasal corticosteroid sprays can be useful in assisting with asthma symptoms in appropriate individuals. Rhinitis medications, however, seem to be less effective than allergen-specific immunotherapy in influencing asthma control over the long term. The use of both subcutaneous and sublingual immunotherapy have been shown to improve asthma symptoms and asthma control, with improvement in outcomes and reduction in asthma exacerbations.

The mainstay of treatment for asthma involves the use of pharmacotherapy to both decrease patient symptoms and to induce long-term control. Medications for the treatment of asthma can be considered in 2 broad categories based on the indications for their use: rescue medications and controller medications. Because the goal of asthma therapy is to achieve control, the strategy of therapy is to treat patients with controller medications and decrease or eliminate the need for them to use rescue medications.

Rescue medications are used by patients to rapidly reverse the symptoms of obstruction, and should be used infrequently for acute need. The most commonly used rescue medication is albuterol, which is a rapidly acting β-2 agonist that functions as a bronchodilator in reducing bronchoconstriction, relaxing smooth muscle, and encouraging improved respiration. Medications such as albuterol are important agents in the treatment of asthma, but do not exert antiinflammatory effects on the airway. As a result, although bronchodilators can improve short-term symptoms, ongoing inflammation will occur, leading to worsening physiologic changes in the lungs and eventually to remodeling. In addition, short-acting bronchodilators have decreasing benefit with repeated use, likely owing to tolerance at the receptor level of central adaptation. These effects can lead to acute failure of response and can be life threatening with frequent use. As such, albuterol and similar medications are best used infrequently and only until control can be achieved with more appropriate agents.

The primary controller medications that are used for the treatment of asthma are inhaled corticosteroids (ICSs). ICSs represent a broad class of medications with anti-inflammatory and immunosuppressive effects, and are considered first-line treatments for the control of asthma. They are the most effective long-term medications for achieving and maintaining asthma control, and newer agents are generally well-tolerated without significant adverse effects. ICSs are not only useful in reducing patient symptoms and in improving disease control, but have been shown to improve pulmonary function with persistent use. They have been shown to reduce asthma morbidity and have been associated with significant decrease in asthma-related mortality.[12]

The most significant adverse effects noted with ICSs are related to hypothalamic–pituitary axis suppression, similar to those seen with systemic corticosteroid medications, but less severe. There seems to be a dose-dependent effect that can be assessed, yet significant consequences are uncommon. Although transient growth suppression in children has been reported with high-dose ICSs, there is not any convincing evidence that there is a sustained effect on adult height. Common side effects also include oral candidiasis and mild to moderate dysphonia, which can be improved by the use of spacers to decrease application of medication to the laryngopharyngeal mucosa.

Another commonly used controller class that is applied in the treatment of asthma is the combination ICS/long-acting β-2 agonist medications. Long-acting β-2 agonists such as salmeterol can be useful in reducing bronchoconstriction, but should not be used alone for the treatment of asthma owing to an increased incidence of asthma-related deaths. When combined with an ICS, these medications can provide excellent asthma control and allow lower doses of ICSs to be prescribed to achieve control. These combination agents are frequently used and have been shown to be safe in the treatment of asthma in adolescents and adults.

Alternate medications can be used for the treatment of asthma in select circumstances. Leukotriene-modifying agents such as montelukast have been shown to improve asthma both alone and in combination with other controller medications. The effect of these medications is inferior in asthma control to ICSs, but they may have specific benefit in aspirin-exacerbated respiratory disease. In addition, they have been shown to be useful in exercise-induced bronchoconstriction. Anticholinergic agents such as ipratropium can also be useful in patients with severe airway obstruction and in patients currently on treatment with β-blockers.

Less frequently used in current practice are older oral bronchodilators such as theophylline and mast cell–inhibiting medications such as cromolyn sodium. Newer monoclonal antibody medications that have select immunomodulatory functions, such as omalizumab, have specific uses in select patients and can reduce the need for systemic steroids in patients with severe disease.

As with the use of all medications, specific patient characteristics and adherence must be assessed in prescribing treatments and in evaluating the response to therapy. As patients achieve control, medications can be adjusted to reduce administered doses and to eliminate the use of multiple medications.

In patients with demonstrated allergic sensitivities, there is substantial evidence that the use of allergen-specific immunotherapy can both facilitate asthma control and improve pulmonary function among atopic patients with asthma. Several studies have shown significant benefit, as reported in a 2010 Cochrane review, which noted improvement in asthma symptoms, reduced pharmacotherapy use, and decreased bronchial hyperresponsiveness.[13] Similar efficacy seems to be present with sublingual immunotherapy as well.[14] Allergen-specific immunotherapy has benefit in the management of patients with asthma and can be considered as an appropriate method in their treatment.

Initiating Therapy

When initiating therapy for asthma, it can be useful to classify the severity and chronicity of the patient's symptoms as a guide to the types and doses of medications to be used. Asthma can be classified into 2 time courses based on the frequency and persistence of symptoms (**Table 1**):

Intermittent
- Symptoms occurring 2 days a week or less;
- Nighttime awakenings 2 days a month or less;
- Use of short-term β-2 agonist 2 days a week or less; and
- No interference with normal activity.

Persistent
- Symptoms occurring more than 2 days a week;
- Nighttime awakenings 3 days a month or more;
- Use of short-term β-2 agonist more than 2 days a week; and
- Some degree of limitations in normal activity.[1]

The 2007 National Heart, Lung, and Blood Institute guidelines further subclassify persistent asthma into 3 levels of severity, based again on the frequency of symptoms and use of rescue medication:

Mild persistent asthma
- Symptoms occurring more than 2 days a week, but not daily;
- Nighttime awakenings 3 or 4 times a month;
- Use of short-term β-2 agonist more than twice a week, but not more than once daily; and
- Minor limitations in normal activity.

Moderate persistent asthma
- Symptoms occurring daily;
- Nighttime awakenings at least once a week, but not nightly;
- Daily use of short-term β-2 agonist; and
- Some clinically significant limitations in normal activity.

Severe persistent asthma
- Symptoms occurring through each day;
- Nighttime awakenings several times weekly;
- Use of short- term β-2 agonist several times daily; and
- Severe limitations in normal activities.

Based on this assessment of severity, therapy can be initiated using guidelines published by the National Heart, Lung, and Blood Institute (**Fig. 1**). For intermittent asthma, short-acting β-2 agonists can be used on an as-needed basis, and can generally control these uncommon symptoms. For persistent asthma, the types and doses of medications used can be determined based on the step care algorithm. In general, therapy

Table 1
Classification of asthma severity

Components of Severity		Classification of Asthma Severity (≥12 Years of Age)			
		Intermittent	Persistent		
			Mild	Moderate	Severe
Impairment	Symptoms	≤2 d/wk	>2 d/wk but not daily	Daily	Throughout the day
Normal FEV₁/FVC: 8–19 y 85%; 20–39 y 80%; 40–59 y 75%; 60–80 y 70%	Nighttime awakenings	<2×/mo	3–4×/mo	>1×/wk but not nightly	Often 7×/wk
	Short-acting beta₂-agonist use for symptom control (not prevention of EIB)	≤2 d/wk	>2 d/wk but not daily, and not more than 1× on any day	Daily	Several times per day
	Interference with normal activity	None	Minor limitation	Some limitation	Extremely limited
	Lung function	• Normal FEV₁ between exacerbations • FEV₁ >80% of predicted • FEV₁/FVC normal	• FEV₁ >80% of predicted • FEV₁/FVC normal	• FEV₁ >60% but <80% of predicted • FEV₁/FVC reduced 5%	• FEV₁ <60% predicted • FEV₁/FVC reduced >5%
Risk	Exacerbations requiring oral systemic corticosteroids	0–1/y[a]	≥2/y[a]		
Recommended step for initiating treatment		Step 1[c]	Step 2[c]	Step 3[b,c]	Step 4 or 5[b,c]

Abbreviations: EIB, exercise-induced bronchoconstriction; FEV₁, forced expiratory volume in 1 second; FVC, forced vital capacity.

[a] Consider severity and interval since last exacerbation. Frequency and severity may fluctuate over time for patients in any severity category Relative annual risk of exacerbations may be related to FEV₁.

[b] And consider a short course of oral systemic corticosteroids.

[c] In 2–6 weeks, evaluate level of asthma control that is achieved and adjust therapy accordingly.

From National Asthma Education and Prevention Program (NAEPP). Guidelines for the Diagnosis and Management of Asthma (EPR-3). Bethesda (MD): National Heart, Lung, and Blood Institute (NHLBI); 2007. Available at: https://www.nhlbi.nih.gov/files/docs/guidelines/asthsumm.pdf. Accessed August 10, 2017.

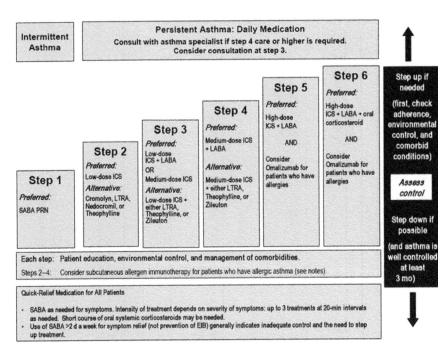

Fig. 1. Stepwise approach to managing asthma based on control. ICS, inhaled corticosteroids; LABA, long-acting β-agonists; LTRA, leukotriene receptor antagonist; SABA, short-acting β. (*From* National Asthma Education and Prevention Program (NAEPP). Guidelines for the Diagnosis and Management of Asthma (EPR-3). Bethesda (MD): National Heart, Lung, and Blood Institute (NHLBI); 2007. Available at: https://www.nhlbi.nih.gov/files/docs/guidelines/asthsumm.pdf. Accessed August 10, 2017.)

can be initiated for moderate persistent asthma in step 3, with a medium-dose ICS or a combination agent of an ICS/long-acting β-2 agonist. Patients with mild persistent asthma may be treated with a low-dose ICS alone at step 2, and patients with severe persistent asthma should be treated at step 4 or higher, with higher doses and combinations of therapeutic agents. In cases of severe persistent asthma, it is wise to have the patient managed by a clinician who specializes in the treatment of patients with asthma.

Once the patient has initiated asthma therapy, the efficacy of that treatment must be assessed periodically to optimize outcome. Whereas patients with severe symptoms should be observed closely and followed on a weekly basis until improved, others can be managed at 4-week intervals, with adjustments in therapeutic intensity based on an assessment of control (**Table 2**). The goal is to facilitate the patient's asthma to being well-controlled, with no limitation in activities and with infrequent symptoms and use of rescue medications. The value of the step care approach to treatment is that by using the National Heart, Lung, and Blood Institute algorithm the clinician can step up or step down therapy by changes in dosing of medications or by adding or removing complementary medications. The clinician should continue to manage patients with the objective of achieving excellent control at the lowest dose and number of medications necessary. Modifications in treatment level can also be made if symptoms worsen owing to factors such as seasonal allergen exposures or concurrent respiratory infections.

Table 2
Components of asthma control

	Components of Control	Classification of Asthma Control (≥12 Years of Age)		
		Well Controlled	Not Well Controlled	Very Poorly Controlled
Impairment	Symptoms	≤2 d/wk	>2 d/wk	Throughout the day
	Nighttime awakenings	≤2×/mo	1–3×/wk	≥4×/wk
	Interference with normal activity	None	Some limitation	Extremely limited
	Short-acting beta-agonist use for symptom control (not prevention of EIB)	≤2 d/wk	>2 d/wk	Several times per day
	FEV_1 or peak flow	>80% predicted/personal best	60%–80% predicted/personal best	<60% predicted/personal best
	Validated Questionnaires			
	ATAQ	0	1–2	3–4
	ACQ	≤0.75	≥1.5	N/A
	ACT	≥20	16–19	≤15
Risk	Exacerbations requiring oral systemic corticosteroids	0–1/y	≥2/y	
		Consider severity and interval since last exacerbation		
	Progressive loss of lung function	Evaluation requires long-term follow-up care		
	Treatment-related adverse effects	Medication side effects can vary in intensity from none to very troublesome and worrisome. The level of intensity does not correlate to specific levels of control but should be considered in the overall assessment of risk.		
Recommended action for treatment		• Maintain current step • Regular follow-ups every 1–6 mo to maintain control • Consider step down if well-controlled for at least 3 mo	• Step up 1 step and • Reevaluate in 2–6 wk • For side effects, consider alternative treatment options.	• Consider short course of oral systemic corticosteroids • Step up 1–2 steps, and • Reevaluate in 2 wk • For side effects, consider alternative treatment options

Abbreviations: ACQ, Asthma Control Questionnaire; ATAQ, Asthma Therapy Assessment Questionnaire; EIB, exercise-induced bronchoconstriction; FEV_1, forced expiratory volume in 1 second; N/A, not applicable.

From National Asthma Education and Prevention Program (NAEPP), Guidelines for the Diagnosis and Management of Asthma (EPR-3). Bethesda (MD): National Heart, Lung, and Blood Institute (NHLBI); 2007. Available at: https://www.nhlbi.nih.gov/files/docs/guidelines/asthsumm.pdf. Accessed August 10, 2017.

SUMMARY

Asthma is a chronic inflammatory disease that will frequently be encountered by otolaryngologists as they manage their patients with upper respiratory diseases. Symptoms such as cough should alert otolaryngologists to consider more broadly the potential role of asthma in the differential diagnosis. It is critical for otolaryngologists to appreciate that patients with allergic rhinitis and chronic rhinosinusitis will often have asthma, and that many of them may not be diagnosed at the time of presentation. Appropriate diagnosis of the patient with asthma, as well as effective treatment for its symptoms, will improve patient function and enhance quality of life.

REFERENCES

1. National Asthma Education and Prevention Program (NAEPP). Guidelines for the diagnosis and management of asthma (EPR-3). Bethesda (MD): National Heart, Lung, and Blood Institute (NHLBI); 2007.
2. Masol M, Fabian D, Holt S, et al. The global burden of asthma: executive summary of the GINA dissemination World Health Organization committee report. Allergy 2004;59:469-78.
3. Krouse JH. The unified airway – conceptual framework. Otolaryngol Clin North Am 2008;41:257-66.
4. Bachert C, van Cauwenberge P, Khaltev N, World Health Organization. Allergic rhinitis and its impact on asthma. In collaboration with the World Health Organization. Executive summary of the workshop report. 7-10 December 1999, Geneva, Switzerland. Allergy 2002;(57):841-55.
5. Fahy JV. Type 2 inflammation in asthma – present in most, absent in many. Nat Rev Immunol 2015;15:57-65.
6. Holgate ST. Pathogenesis of asthma. Clin Exp Allergy 2008;38:872-97.
7. Bachert C, Vignola AM, Gevaert P, et al. Allergic rhinitis, rhinosinusitis, and asthma: one airway disease. Immunol Allergy Clin North Am 2004;24:19-43.
8. Busse WW, Lemanske RF Jr. Asthma. N Engl J Med 2001;344:350-62.
9. Settipane GA, Greisner WA 3rd, Settipane RJ. Natural history of asthma: a 23-year followup of college students. Ann Allergy Asthma Immunol 2000;84:499-503.
10. Reddel HK, Bateman ED, Becker A, et al. A summary of the new GINA strategy: a roadmap to asthma control. Eur Respir J 2015;46:622-39.
11. Mener DJ, Lin SY. Improvement and prevention of asthma with concomitant treatment of allergic rhinitis and allergen-specific therapy. Int Forum Allergy Rhinol 2015;5:S45-50.
12. Suissa S, Ernst P, Benayoun S, et al. Low-dose inhaled corticosteroids and the prevention of death from asthma. N Engl J Med 2000;343:332-6.
13. Abramson MJ, Puy RM, Weiner JM. Injection allergen immunotherapy for asthma. Cochrane Database Syst Rev 2010;(8):CD00186.
14. Passalacqua G, Durham SR. Allergic rhinitis and its impact on asthma update: allergen immunotherapy. J Allergy Clin Immunol 2007;119:881-91.

The Role of Allergy in Chronic Rhinosinusitis

Ashleigh A. Halderman, MD*, Laura J. Tully, MD

KEYWORDS

- Chronic rhinosinusitis • Chronic rhinosinusitis with nasal polyps
- Chronic rhinosinusitis without nasal polyps • Allergic fungal rhinosinusitis • Allergies
- Allergic rhinitis

KEY POINTS

- Allergy and CRS often co-occur but a direct link establishing causality has not been identified.
- There is far more overlap in the pathophysiology of allergy and chronic rhinosinusitis with nasal polyps and allergic fungal rhinosinusitis than there is between allergy and chronic rhinosinusitis without nasal polyps.
- Seasonal allergies do not appear to contribute to rhinosinusitis in any form; however, perennial allergies may.
- Weak evidence exists for the use of immunotherapy in CRS with significant limitations of current available studies.

INTRODUCTION

Chronic rhinosinusitis (CRS), both with and without polyps, has an estimated prevalence of 4.9% ± 0.2% (or 490 in 10,000 people) in the United States.[1,2] The prevalence of allergic rhinitis (AR) in the general population is between 10% and 30%.[3,4] Some studies have shown that patients with sinusitis have a higher incidence of positive allergy skin prick tests (SPTs) than the general population,[5–7] other studies do not support this.[8,9] Likely, the 2 disease processes often coexist, but the data supporting the role or association of allergy and CRS are mixed.[10] This is not surprising because the definitions of both allergy and CRS can vary widely between studies, introducing an inherently heterogeneous study population over the whole of the literature. Furthermore, there is some evidence that the type of allergy (seasonal vs perennial) also needs to be taken into consideration because studies have shown that seasonal allergies do not seem to predispose a person to sinusitis but perennial allergies might.[7,11,12]

Department of Otolaryngology–Head and Neck Surgery, University of Texas Southwestern Medical Center, 5303 Harry Hines Boulevard, Dallas, TX 75390, USA
* Corresponding author.
E-mail address: ashleigh.halderman@utsouthwestern.edu

Otolaryngol Clin N Am 50 (2017) 1077–1090
http://dx.doi.org/10.1016/j.otc.2017.08.003
0030-6665/17/© 2017 Elsevier Inc. All rights reserved.

CRS is likely a multifactorial disease with environmental, immunologic, microbacterial, genetic, and, possibly, allergic factors at play. Over time, a complex picture of the molecular and cellular mechanisms underlying CRS has begun to emerge and has led to the conceptualization of CRS endotypes. Endotypes represent subtypes of CRS defined by unique pathophysiologic mechanisms and biomarkers.[13] Until these endotypes have been better characterized and understood, the recognition of specific clinical CRS phenotypes and consideration of them as having different underlying pathophysiologies are of the utmost importance. As such, this review considers the role of allergy in the following disease states: CRS without nasal polyps (CRSsNP), CRS with nasal polyps (CRSwNP), and allergic fungal rhinosinusitis (AFRS).

CHRONIC RHINOSINUSITIS WITHOUT NASAL POLYPS

Diagnostic criteria[14] for CRSsNP include the presence of 2 or more of the following symptoms for at least 12 weeks:

- Nasal drainage (anterior rhinorrhea or postnasal drip)
- Nasal obstruction/congestion
- Hyposmia or anosmia
- Facial pain/pressure

And in addition

- Lack of nasal polyps

And either

- Evidence of paranasal sinus inflammation on CT
- Evidence of purulence coming from the sinuses or ostiomeatal complex on endoscopy

T cells are thought to be a crucial driver for the inflammatory cascade observed in most CRSsNP cases, which is generally marked by elevated levels of tumor necrosis factor (TNF)-α, interleukin (IL)-1β, IL-5, and IL-8.[15] As discussed previously, the exact underlying cause of CRSsNP is not completely understood and is likely multifactorial. Unfortunately, no controlled studies on the role of allergy in the pathophysiology of CRSsNP have been performed; therefore, only associations, such as the following, can be made.

A proposed mechanism by which allergy leads to the development of sinusitis is allergy-induced mucosal inflammation leading to ostial obstruction. Ostial obstruction in turn may promote an environment for bacterial overgrowth and/or perpetuation of inflammation. Certainly, in the nasal passages, IgE-mediated degranulation of mast cells leads to mucosal edema. Whether this same process occurs in the paranasal sinuses is less clear. In 1 study, Baroody and colleagues[16] performed a nasal allergen challenge in patients confirmed allergic on SPT followed by nasal and maxillary sinus lavage. After nasal challenge, they found a significant increase in the levels of histamine, albumin, and number of eosinophils in maxillary sinus lavage. These levels were smaller in magnitude than nasal passage levels, but this study did demonstrate a parallel inflammatory response within the maxillary sinuses.[16] Another study biopsied the inferior turbinate of patients confirmed to be allergic on SPT who were prone to sinusitis (defined as at least 2 sinus infections per year confirmed on maxillary puncture) to controls. Biopsies were taken in each patient during an acute viral upper respiratory infection and later during convalescence. The allergic patients prone to sinusitis were found to have significantly elevated T cells and lower levels of mast cells in convalescence compared with controls.[17] This was not seen in allergic patients not prone to sinusitis.[17] The investigators postulated that this delayed accumulation of intraepithelial T cells could indicate a prolonged inflammatory reaction in those patients prone to sinusitis.[17] Certainly, given the evidence of T-cell–mediated inflammation in CRSsNP, this is an intriguing finding.

Studies have shown that AR and nasal eosinophilia can impair nasal mucociliary clearance.[18,19] Impaired ciliary function and mucociliary clearance are often observed in CRSsNP as well. Cilia from patients with CRSsNP have demonstrated a blunted response to substances that typically stimulate cilia in healthy controls.[20,21] Furthermore, the underlying chronic inflammation in CRSsNP has been shown to cause ciliary loss or abnormalities over time.[22] Based on this evidence, it is possible that the ciliary dysfunction observed in CRSsNP could be exacerbated further in those patients with concurrent AR and that allergy contributes to the disease process in this way.

Many studies have investigated a connection between allergy and sinusitis based on clinical evidence, but few have done so in a pure CRSsNP population. Most studies have applied the generic term, *sinusitis*, to their patient populations, and on further reading, it becomes clear that their definition or criteria for sinusitis best fit the current criteria for acute or recurrent acute sinusitis rather than CRSsNP. Moreover, many studies using the term, *chronic sinusitis*, include both polyp and nonpolyp patients in the same study group. This is problematic, because CRSsNP and CRSwNP are now understood to differ significantly in both clinical and pathophysiologic features. It is perhaps for this reason that several older studies reported a much higher prevalence of allergic patients in their CRS cohort than expected, ranging from 36.2% to 84% prevalence.[6,7,23] As discussed later, allergy is possibly more prevalent in CRSwNP compared with CRSsNP and, therefore, it is conceivable these numbers were skewed with the inclusion of polyp patients. These same studies all found either a significant association of allergy with CRS or that the presence of allergy was associated with increased severity of disease.[6,7,23] Again, these findings would likely be altered by the inclusion of polyp patients.

Applying the current diagnostic criteria of symptoms for at least 12 weeks and an absence of polyps, 3 cross-sectional study comparing allergic patients to nonallergic patients were identified. Kirtsreesakul and Ruttanphol[24] recruited patients with at least 3 months of nasal symptoms and tested them via SPT for allergy. They compared the findings on conventional sinus radiography and nasal endoscopy for SPT-positive and SPT-negative patients. Although they found no significant differences on endoscopy, they did discover that allergic patients were 2.8-times more likely to have abnormalities on plain films than were nonallergic patients ($P<.001$).[24] Conventional sinus radiography has largely been abandoned due to high numbers of false-positive and false-negative results and is a shortcoming of this study. No significant differences were found on nasal endoscopy between the groups.[24] Berettini and colleagues[25] compared 40 patients with perennial AR to healthy controls and found a significant increase in the prevalence of sinusitis on CT scans in the allergic group ($P = .017$). Similarly, Ramadan and colleagues[26] showed atopic patients had higher mean Lund-Mackay scores (LMS) than nonatopic patients ($P = .03$). Together, these studies all provide evidence that patients with allergy and CRSsNP may have more severe clinical disease and possibly a higher prevalence of sinusitis than nonallergic patients suggesting a contribution or association of allergy to CRSsNP.

Where these supported a contribution or association of the 2 diseases, several other studies have failed. Robinson and colleagues[27] assessed for atopy via in vitro testing in 193 patients with CRSsNP and CRSwNP. They found a significantly increased prevalence of atopy in the CRSsNP compared with the CRSwNP group (32.3% vs 27.5%;

$P = .05$); however, they failed to show a significant impact of atopy on Sino-Nasal Outcome Test (SNOT)-20 overall scores, Lund symptom scores, LMS, or need for revision surgery. Similarly, multiple other studies have failed to show significant differences in LMS between allergic and nonallergic CRSsNP patients.[28–31] Gelincik and colleagues[28] further demonstrated that CRS symptom scores ($P = .045$) and global CRS scores ($P = .01$) were actually significantly higher in nonallergic rhinitis patients compared with those with AR in their CRS population. The only significant difference on nasal endoscopy was an increased rate of nasal purulence observed in AR patients ($P = .002$) for which no explanation was given.[28]

With such conflicting results in the literature, it is difficult to come to any conclusions on the role of allergy in CRSsNP. What does become clear is the potential for future well-designed studies to either establish a role or to determine one does not exist. Regardless, patients with co-occurring allergies and CRSsNP should be treated for both as per the recommendations of available clinical guidelines.

CHRONIC RHINOSINUSITIS WITH POLYPS

CRSwNP reportedly occurs in 0.5% to 4.3% of the population.[32] The prevalence tends to increase with age and the disease occurs more often in men. The diagnostic criteria for CRSwNP are the same as those for CRSsNP with one important difference, polyps must be present.[14] It is generally more recalcitrant than CRSsNP with a reported 38% to 69% of revision endoscopic sinus surgery cases attributed to CRSwNP.[30,33,34]

Similar to allergy, CRSwNP is characterized by helper T-cell type 2 (T_H2) cytokine-mediated inflammation (including elevated levels of IL-5 and IL-13), eosinophilic inflammation, and elevated IgE.[35,36] In 80% of patients with CRSwNP, polyps are characterized by eosinophilia and an up-regulation of IL-5.[37,38] Patients with polyps often demonstrate both local production of mucosal IgE and elevated levels of circulating IgE.[38–40] Polyclonal IgE antibodies from polyps have been shown to be capable of activating mast cells on allergen challenge ex vivo.[40] It has been theorized that with continual exposure to inhaled allergens in sensitized patients, these polyclonal IgE antibodies contribute to persistent inflammation in CRSwNP.[40] Finally, IL-13 has been both implicated in the T_H2-driven inflammation seen in CRSwNP and the pathology of allergic diseases.[41] From a pathophysiologic standpoint, allergy and CRSwNP seem to share a fair amount of overlap.

As far as an association between allergy and CRSwNP, several studies have demonstrated an increased prevalence for perennial allergies in patients with CRSwNP compared with controls, with reports varying between 45% to 77.4%.[12,29,42–44] Additionally, 2 studies showed a strong association between perennial allergies and CRSwNP with odds ratios of 2.69 and 6.0 described.[12,44] In both studies, there was a strong association between dust mite sensitivity and CRSwNP, which has also been described by Asero and Bottazzi.[43] Other studies have shown a high proportion of CRSwNP patients to be sensitized to molds.[12,43,44] In 2 separate studies, Asero and Bottazzi showed a significantly higher prevalence of sensitivity to *Candida albicans* in CRSwNP patients compared with controls with a prevalence of 40% versus 11% ($P<.001$) shown in 1 study[42] and 44% versus 1% ($P<.001$) in another.[43] Tan and colleagues[29] reviewed their population of CRS patients who failed medical therapy and went on to have surgery. They found a trend toward increasing atopy rates in CRSwNP and that their CRSwNP patients had a significantly higher mean number of positive SPT results compared with the CRSsNP group ($P = .033$) and rhinitis group ($P<.01$). All of this taken together supports a possible role, if not an association, of perennial allergies with CRSwNP.

Few studies have looked at the clinical impact of allergies on patients with CRSwNP. Kirtsreesakul[45] performed one of the few available clinical studies where they compared various outcomes of a therapy for budesonide nasal spray on SPT-positive and SPT-negative CRSwNP patients. Overall, they found after 6 weeks of treatment, the SPT-positive group saw less improvement in polyp size, expiratory peak flows, and overall efficacy score than did the SPT-negative group.[45] These findings suggest that among polyp patients, those with concurrent allergy may do worse or be less responsive to standard therapy. Unfortunately, there are few additional data to support these findings.

Regarding seasonal allergies and CRSwNP, in 1 study by Asero and Bottazzi,[43] an increased prevalence of sensitivity on SPT to at least 1 seasonal allergen was documented in their control patients (84%) versus CRSwNP patients (60%) ($P<.005$). Furthermore, many others have demonstrated a lack of increased prevalence of seasonal allergies in CRSwNP patients.[12,29,42] Keith and colleagues[46] demonstrated that seasonal allergy exposure in patients with nasal polyps does not enhance the level of expression of disease as determined by symptom scores and concentrations of eosinophils, eosinophilic cationic protein, and albumin both in and out of ragweed season. Therefore, at this time, based on the available literature, it seems that evidence for an association between seasonal allergies and CRSwNP is lacking.

Contradicting the findings of those reviewed previously is a study by Gorgulu and colleagues.[47] In their population of patients with CRSwNP who had undergone prior sinus surgery, the prevalence of allergy was 25% compared with 28% in controls. Additionally, in a regression model, allergy was not determined a significant risk factor for developing nasal polyps.[47] Other studies showed a similar prevalence of allergy in CRSwNP with a range between 19.5% and 35%.[36,48,49] This is still higher than the general population but is considerably lower than others who have reported a prevalence of allergy in CRSwNP patients requiring surgery as high as 85.5%.[29]

Numerous studies have failed to show an impact of allergy on either the severity of CRSwNP or the response to treatment. In 2 separate studies, Bonfils and colleagues[48] compared patients with CRSwNP and allergy to those without allergy. In 1 study, after 1 year of treatment with saline washes, intranasal steroids, and oral steroids, there were no significant differences in changes in symptom scores between the groups. Additionally, there was no significant difference in the consumption or use of nasal or oral steroids between the 2 groups.[48] This was again demonstrated in a later study where quantities of oral and nasal steroids were consumed at similar rates regardless of allergy status over a mean 5.8-year follow-up period.[49]

Erbek and colleagues[50] evaluated multiple clinical parameters as well as serum markers in CRSwNP patients with and without allergy. As expected, they demonstrated significantly higher serum total eosinophil and IgE counts in allergic patients compared with nonallergic patients ($P<.05$). They discovered a correlation between blood total eosinophil count and LMS in allergic patients with nasal polyps ($P = .005$).[50] Serum total IgE levels did not correlate, however, with LMS and neither IgE nor eosinophil levels seemed to have an impact on any other parameters of disease severity.[50] Additionally, the diagnosis of allergy was not associated with polyp size, LMS, or symptom scores.[50] Other studies also failed to demonstrate an association between the presence of allergy and either more severe symptom scores or polyp grade in CRSwNP.[48,49]

Despite conflicting reports in the literature, a few conclusions about allergy and CRSwNP can be made. The prevalence of allergy in patients with CRSwNP is higher than that of the general population and may be higher than in CRSsNP. The underlying pathophysiology with T_H2-skewed inflammation, eosinophilia, and elevated IgE seen in many patients with CRSwNP significantly overlaps and is similar in many ways to the pathophysiology of allergy. From this, it could easily be surmised that the processes may be related and/or interdependent on each another. Certainly, the evidence of tissue polyclonal IgE-activating mast cells in response to allergen exposure is compelling. Clinical evidence supporting a meaningful contribution of allergy to CRSwNP is, however, much weaker.

IMMUNOTHERAPY AND CHRONIC SINUSITIS

There is a surprising paucity of information regarding the use of immunotherapy (IT) in the treatment of CRSsNP and CRSwNP. A systematic review by DeYoung and colleagues[51] identified and reviewed 7 studies on the effect of IT in patients with CRS (patients were not always separated into CRSsNP and CRSwNP groups), none of which was a randomized controlled trial. Two studies compared symptom scores in atopic CRS patients treated with IT compared with those whose atopy was medically managed. Both studies showed significantly improved symptom scores in the IT groups[52,53]; however, in 1 study, there were significant differences in various baseline symptoms between the groups, which could have skewed the results,[52] and baseline scores were not included to assure equality between the groups in the second.[53]

A few studies reported on endoscopic outcomes in CRS patients on IT. One study found a decrease in inferior turbinate hypertrophy in the IT group compared with the control group,[52] and a second study described less middle meatus closure and synechiae formation after surgery in their IT group compared with controls.[54] The effect of IT on polyp recurrence after surgery was studied by Nishioka and colleagues.[54] They reported a recurrence in 35.3% of atopic CRSwNP patients on IT compared with 40% of atopic CRSwNP not treated with IT. Unfortunately, their control group only consisted of 5 patients meaning this study was underpowered. Finally, Schlenter and Man[53] compared CT scores in atopic CRS patients treated with IT to those who were not and found that the IT group showed a 40% improvement in their radiographic score compared with 27% in the control group.

In their systematic review, DeYoung and colleagues[51] concluded that there was weak evidence in support of the use of IT in atopic patients with CRS. Overall, the strength of the available literature is limited due to a lack of randomization and blinding in studies conducted on the use of IT in patients with CRS. Additionally, it has been well established that IT does improve symptoms of AR,[55] which share a considerable overlap with symptoms of CRS. Whether IT modulates the disease process of CRSsNP and CRSwNP has yet to be determined.

ALLERGIC FUNGAL RHINOSINUSITIS

AFRS is a noninvasive, eosinophilic, recurrent form of polypoid rhinosinusitis that affects immunocompetent hosts. It is the most common form of fungal sinusitis in the United States, with the highest prevalence in the southeast and south central portions.[55] The higher prevalence in this region of the United States is thought to be because of the warm, humid environment, which may increase a person's exposure to fungi; however, studies have failed to clearly demonstrate a correlation between mold counts and incidence of AFRS.[56] The most common fungi isolated in AFRS are dematiaceous fungi, including *Alternaria, Bipolaris, Drechslera, Curvularia*, and *Exserohilum* species.[57] Patients with AFRS tend to be diagnosed at a younger age than patients with CRSwNP and CRSsNP, with the average age of diagnosis at 28 years versus 48 and 43 years, respectively.[58] Additionally, it has been shown that African Americans with AFRS are diagnosed at an even younger age and have more severe disease at presentation than Caucasians.[59] Retrospective studies have demonstrated an association between AFRS and low socioeconomic status.[58,60,61] The current accepted management of AFRS is with primary endoscopic sinus surgery followed by postoperative oral corticosteroids.[14] Despite this, the recurrent rates are high, and AFRS is considered a chronic condition.

In 1983 Katzenstein and colleagues[62] documented a case series of patients with noninvasive aspergillus sinusitis, nasal polyps, and allergic mucin on histology, which they termed, *allergic aspergillus sinusitis*. The disease was thought to be related to allergic bronchopulmonary aspergillosis. In 1991, Manning and colleagues[63] demonstrated that other fungal species were more commonly isolated than *Aspergillus* in these patients, including *Bipolaris, Alternaria,* and *Curvularia* and termed the disease, *allergic fungal sinusitis*. In 1994, Bent and Kuhn[64] developed 5 diagnostic criteria for allergic fungal sinusitis, including

- Type 1 hypersensitivity confirmed by history, skin tests, or serology
- Nasal polyposis
- Eosinophilic mucin without fungal invasion
- Characteristic CT signs
  - Increased density of material within the sinus cavities seen in **Fig. 1**
  - Expansion or erosion of the paranasal sinus bony walls seen in **Fig. 2**
- Positive fungal stain

The disease process was initially named allergic fungal sinusitis but has been broadened to AFRS to signify the involvement of both the nasal passages and paranasal sinuses.[65] Some investigators have recommended positive fungal culture instead of positive fungal stain as an alternative diagnostic criterion for AFRS; however, fungal culture has been shown to have variable sensitivity, and, therefore, fungal stain remains the more reliable indicator of AFRS at this time.[14,66]

The pathophysiologic basis of AFRS is thought to be secondary to a type I hypersensitivity (IgE-mediated) inflammatory response to extramucosal fungi within the nasal cavity and paranasal sinuses.[67,68] The theory regarding an IgE-mediated immune response to fungal antigens was based on the proposed mechanisms behind

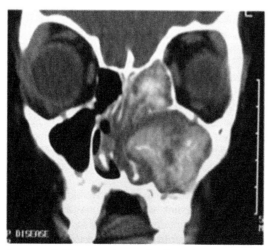

Fig. 1. Noncontrast coronal CT scan demonstrating characteristic CT signs, including increased density of material within the sinus cavities.

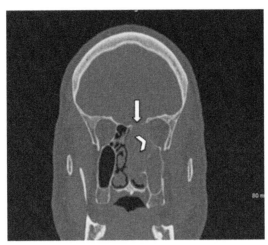

Fig. 2. Noncontrast coronal CT scan demonstrating erosion of the skull base (*arrow*) and the lamina papyracea (*arrowhead*).

allergic bronchopulmonary aspergillosis.[66] Fungal allergy is defined by the presence of elevated levels of fungal-specific IgE or positive SPT to fungal antigens.[69]

In a large series, more than 90% of patients with AFRS had a type I hypersensitivity reaction observed via skin testing against aspergillin antigen.[70] This is compared with a rate of 10% to 30% in the general population. The significantly increased prevalence of fungal allergy in patients with AFRS compared with controls suggests a likely contribution of allergy to this disease process. Additionally, patients with AFRS have demonstrated elevated serum total IgE and fungal-specific IgE compared with patients with CRSsNP and CRSwNP and with normal controls.[71] The serum IgE levels in patients with AFRS often exceeds 1000 IU/mL, whereas less than 180 IU/mL is considered normal.[58] It has also been shown that increased serum-specific IgE levels to fungal allergens correlate with clinical disease severity and recurrence.[14] Hutcheson and colleagues[71] demonstrated that total serum IgE and IgG anti-*Alternaria* antibodies are significantly elevated in AFRS compared with CRSwNP, indicating heightened fungal immune responses in AFRS patients. Furthermore, in the same study, Western immunoblotting showed fungal-specific IgE as well as increased total IgE in AFRS patients, reinforcing the existence of an allergic component in the pathophysiology of AFRS.[71] It has also been demonstrated that local antigen-specific IgE levels are significantly increased in AFRS patients compared with CRSsNP and CRSwNP patients and are absent in controls.[72] Additionally, several studies have demonstrated elevation of fungal-specific IgE within the sinonasal mucosa of patients with AFRS, which correlates with sinonasal eosinophilia.[73,74] Specifically, Collins and colleagues[75] demonstrated that patients with AFRS were significantly more likely to have fungal-specific IgE in sinus mucin than patients with CRSwNP. These findings support the possibility of local sinonasal IgE production in the pathophysiology of AFRS stemming from an allergy to fungi.

Further details of the unique underlying pathophysiology of AFRS emerged through several immunohistochemical studies, which demonstrated that eosinophils and CD8 cells are more abundant in nasal mucosa of patients with AFRS than in patients with CRSsNP or CRSwNP.[76–78] It is theorized that these fungal-activated eosinophils are capable of inducing proliferation of CD4 and CD8 cells resulting in the production of a fungal-specific Th2 immune response.

Although there is a lack of randomized, controlled studies with regard to IT in the management of AFRS, uncontrolled studies do support IT as an adjunctive medical treatment after surgical management in AFRS.[79–84] Additionally, a small case series using sublingual IT as an adjunctive medical therapy found improvement in LMS as well as decreased total serum IgE levels in patients with AFRS.[85] The low-level evidence suggests that there is a trend toward improved outcomes with IT and that IT may reduce inflammation and steroid requirements in AFRS patients.[58] A recent retrospective study evaluating the efficacy of omalizumab, a humanized monoclonal anti-IgE antibody, in the treatment of AFRS demonstrated clinical improvement in SNOT-22 scores and endoscopic scores.[86] By demonstrating improvement with IT and anti-IgE antibody treatment, these studies further support a role of allergy in the pathophysiology and clinical manifestations of AFRS.

In 1 long-term study comparing AFRS patients treated with IT to those without, Folker and colleagues[87] showed less severe symptoms in patients treated with IT ($P = .002$) as well as significantly lower Kupferberg endoscopic staging. At a second time point 4 years later, there were no difference in symptom scores or endoscopic staging between IT and non-IT groups.[88] Additionally, there was no significant difference in the number of sinus surgeries or use of oral antibiotics between the 2 groups over an average 82-month follow-up period.[88] This study has one of the longest follow-up periods and therefore suggests that AFRS patients treated with IT may initially do better in some parameters, but that this added benefit decreases over time.

Not all studies have supported a role for allergy in the pathophysiology of AFRS, and some investigators have described alternative pathways. For example, Pant and colleagues[69] demonstrated elevated fungal-specific IgG levels in patients with AFRS compared with controls, which suggests contribution from an alternative pathway not modulated by IgE. Additionally, in a large case series of AFRS patients, 33% of patients did not have positive immediate hypersensitivity skin test responses to the fungal species associated with AFRS[89], and Saravanan and colleagues[70] demonstrated that 10% of patients with AFRS were nonreactive to skin testing for aspergillin antigen. Based on these findings, some investigators hypothesize that immune mechanisms other than fungal allergy play a role in the pathogenesis of AFRS. In light of these studies, some investigators support creating a new diagnostic category for patients who meet all Bent and Kuhn diagnostic criteria for AFRS but who do not have evidence of type 1 hypersensitivity to fungal antigens, a disease process referred to as eosinophilic fungal rhinosinusitis.[58]

Despite the data demonstrating elevated levels of fungal-specific IgG and other nonallergic mechanisms, such as bacterial superinfection, there is a tremendous amount of data to support the presence of and possible role for allergy and IgE-driven inflammation in a large proportion of AFRS patients. It is possible that like other forms of CRS, AFRS also has multiple unique endotypes that have yet to be fully characterized.

SUMMARY

Due to a large degree of heterogeneity in the definition of both allergy and CRS, the literature investigating a potential role for allergy in CRS is mixed and often contradictory. Furthermore, several studies were conducted prior to the current accepted distinction of CRS subtypes, such as CRSsNP, CRSwNP, and AFRS. Although no definitive statements in regard to the role allergy plays in CRS can be made, this review has hopefully identified an area in which future studies could greatly advance understanding, with the potential to improve patient care and outcomes.

REFERENCES

1. Bhattacharyya N. Incremental health care utilization and expenditures for chronic rhinosinusitis in the United States. Ann Otol Rhinol Laryngol 2011;120:423–7.
2. Bhattacharyya N. Incremental healthcare utilization and expenditures for allergic rhinitis in the United States. Laryngoscope 2011;121:1830–3.
3. Wallace DV, Dykewicz MS, Bernstein DI, et al. The diagnosis and management of rhinitis; an updated practice parameter. Joint task force on practice parameters. J Allergy Clin Immunol 2008;122(2 Suppl):S1–84.
4. Fougard T. Allergy and allergy-like symptoms in 1,050 medical students. Allergy 1991;46:20–6.
5. Rachelefsky GS, Siegel SC, Katz RM, et al. Chronic sinusitis in children. J Allergy Clin Immunol 1991;87:219.
6. Emanuel IA, Shah SB. Chronic rhinosinusitis: allergy and sinus computed tomography relationships. Otolaryngol Head Neck Surg 2000;123:687–91.
7. Gutman M, Torres A, Keen KJ, et al. Prevalence of allergy in patients with chronic rhinosinusitis. Otolaryngol Head Neck Surg 2004;130:545–52.
8. Iwens P, Clement PAR. Sinusitis in allergic patients. Rhinology 1994;32:65–7.
9. Nguyen KL, Corbett ML, Garcia DP, et al. Chronic sinusitis among pediatric patients with chronic respiratory complaints. J Allergy Clin Immunol 1993;92: 824–30.
10. Wilson KF, McMains C, Orlandi RF. The association between allergy and chronic rhinosinusitis with and without nasal polyposis: an evidence-based review with recommendations. Int Forum Allergy Rhinol 2014;4:93–103.
11. Melen I, Ivarsson A, Schrewelius C. Ostial function in allergic rhinitis. Acta Otolaryngol 1992;(Suppl 492):82–5.
12. Houser SM, Keen KJ. The role of allergy and smoking in chronic rhinosinusitis and polyposis. Laryngoscope 2008;118:1521–7.
13. Akdis CA, Bachert C, Cingi C, et al. Endotypes and phenotypes of chronic rhinosinusitis; A PRACTALL document of the European academy of allergy and clinical immunology and the American academy of allergy, asthma and immunology. J Allergy Clin Immunol 2013;131:1479–90.
14. Orlandi RR, Kingdom TT, Hwang PH, et al. International consensus statement on allergy and rhinology: rhinosinusitis. Int Forum Allergy Rhinol 2016;6:S22–209.
15. Lennard CM, Mann EA, Sun LL, et al. Interleukin-1 beta, interleukin-5, interleukin-6, interleukin-8, and tumor necrosis factor-alpha in chronic sinusitis: response to systemic corticosteroids. Am J Rhinol 2000;14:367–73.
16. Baroody FM, Mucha SM, deTineo M, et al. Nasal challenge with allergen leads to maxillary sinus inflammation. J Allergy Clin Immunol 2008;121:1126–32.
17. Alho OP, Karttunen R, Karttaunen TJ. Nasal mucosa in natural colds: effects of allergic rhinitis and susceptibility to recurrent sinusitis. Clin Exp Immunol 2008; 121:1126–32.
18. Schuhl JF. Nasal mucociliary clearance in perennial rhinitis. J Investig Allergol Clin Immunol 1995;5:333–6.
19. Davidson AE, Miller SD, Settipane RJ, et al. Delayed nasal mucociliary clearance in patients with nonallergic rhinitis and nasal eosinophilia. Allergy Proc 1992;13: 81–4.
20. Chen B, Shaari J, Claire SE, et al. Altered ciliary dynamics in chronic rhinosinusitis. Am J Rhinol 2006;20:325–9.
21. Davis SS, Illum L. Absorption enhancers for nasal drug delivery. Clin Pharmacokinet 2003;42:1107–28.

22. Gudis D, Zhao KQ, Cohen NA. Acquired cilia dysfunction in chronic rhinosinusitis. Am J Rhinol Allergy 2012;26:1–6.
23. Dursun E, Korkmaz H, Eryilmaz A, et al. Clinical predictors of long-term success after endoscopic sinus surgery. Otolaryngol Head Neck Surg 2003;129:526–31.
24. Kirtsreesakul V, Ruttanaphol S. The relationship between allergy and rhinosinusitis. Rhinology 2008;46:204–8.
25. Berettini S, Carabelli A, Sellari-Franceschini S, et al. Perennial allergic rhinitis and chronic sinusitis: correlation with rhinologic risk factor. Allergy 1999;54:242–8.
26. Ramadan HH, Fornelli R, Ortiz AO, et al. Correlation of allergy and severity of sinus disease. Am J Rhinol 1999;13:345–7.
27. Robinson S, Douglas R, Wormald PJ. The relationship between atopy and chronic rhinosinusitis. Am J Rhinol 2006;20:625–8.
28. Gelincik A, Buyukozturk S, Aslan I, et al. Allergic vs nonallergic rhinitis: which is more predisposing to chronic rhinosinusitis? Ann Allergy Asthma Immunol 2008; 101:18–22.
29. Tan BK, Zirkle W, Chandra R, et al. Atopic profile of patients failing medical therapy for chronic rhinosinusitis. Int Forum Allergy Rhinol 2011;1:88–94.
30. Pearlman AN, Chandra RK, Chag D, et al. Relationships between severity of chronic rhinosinusitis and nasal polyposis, asthma, and atopy. Am J Rhinol Allergy 2009;23:145–8.
31. Brooks CD, Kuperstock JE, Rubin SJ, et al. The association of allergic sensitization with radiographic sinus opacification. Am J Rhinol Allergy 2017;31:12–5.
32. Fokkens W, Lund VJ, Mullol J, et al. European position paper on rhinosinusitis and nasal polyps. Rhinol Suppl 2007;20:1–36.
33. Batra PS, Tong L, Citardi MJ. Analysis of comorbidities and objective parameters in refractory chronic rhinosinusitis. Laryngoscope 2013;123(Suppl 7):S1–11.
34. Soler ZM, Sauer DA, Mace J, et al. Relationship between clinical measures and histopathologic findings in chronic rhinosinusitis. Otolaryngol Head Neck Surg 2009;141:454–61.
35. Bachert C, Gevaert P, Holtappels G, et al. Total and specific IgE in nasal polyps is related to local eosinophilic inflammation. J Allergy Clin Immunol 2001;107(4): 607–14.
36. Voegels RL, Santoro P, Butugan O, et al. Nasal polyposis and allergy: is there a correlation? Am J Rhinol 2001;15:9–14.
37. Bachert C, Gevaert P, Holtappels G, et al. Nasal polyposis: from cytokines to growth. Am J Rhinol 2000;14(5):279–90.
38. Bachert C, Wagenmann M, Hauser U, et al. IL-5 synthesis is upregulated in human nasal polyp tissue. J Allergy Clin Immunol 1997;99(6 Pt 1):837–42.
39. Sheahan P, Ahn CN, Harvey RJ, et al. Local IgE production in nonatopic nasal polyposis. J Otolaryngol Head Neck Surg 2010;39(1):45–51.
40. Zhang N, Holtappels G, Gevaert P, et al. Mucosal tissue polyclonal IgE is functional in response to allergen and SEB. Allergy 2011;66(1):141–8.
41. Izhura K, Arima K, Yasunaga S. IL-4 and IL-13: their pathological roles in allergic disease and their potential in developing new therapies. Curr Drug Targets Inflamm Allergy 2002;1:263–9.
42. Asero R, Bottazzi G. Hypersenstivity to molds in patients with nasal polyposis: a clinical study. J Allergy Clin Immunol 2000;105:186–8.
43. Asero R, Bottazzi G. Nasal polyposis: a study of its association with airborne allergen hypersensitivity. Ann Allergy Asthma Immunol 2001;86:283–5.
44. Pumhirun P, Limitlaohapanth C, Wasuwat P. Role of allergy in nasal polyps of Thai patients. Asian Pac J Allergy Immunol 1999;17:13–5.

45. Kirtsreesakul V. Role of allergy in therapeutic response of nasal polyps. Asian Pac J Allergy Immunol 2002;20:141–6.

46. Keith PK, Conway M, Evans S, et al. Nasal polyps: effects of seasonal allergen exposure. J Allergy Clin Immunol 1994;93:567–74.

47. Gorgulu O, Ozdemir S, Canbolat EP, et al. Analysis of the roles of smoking and allergy in nasal polyposis. Ann Otol Rhinol Laryngol 2012;121:615–9.

48. Bonfils P, Avan P, Malinvaud D. Influence of allergy on the symptoms and treatment of nasal polyposis. Acta Otolaryngol 2006;126:839–44.

49. Bonfils P, Malinvaud D. Influence of allergy in patients with nasal polyposis after endoscopic sinus surgery. Acta Otolaryngol 2008;128:186–92.

50. Erbek S, Topal O, Cakmak O. The role of allergy in the severity of nasal polyposis. Am J Rhinol 2007;21:686–90.

51. DeYoung K, Wentzel JL, Schlosser RJ, et al. Systematic review of immunotherapy for chronic rhinosinusitis. Am J Rhinol Allergy 2014;28:145–50.

52. Asakura K, Kojima T, Shirasaki H, et al. Evaluation of the effects of antigen specific immunotherapy on chronic sinusitis in children with allergy. Auris Nasus Larynx 1990;17:33–8.

53. Schlenter WW, Man WJ. Operative therapy for chronic sinusitis-results with allergic and non-allergic patients. Laryngol Rhinol Otol 1983;62:284–8.

54. Nishioka GJ, Cook PR, Davis WE, et al. Immunotherapy in patients undergoing functional endoscopic sinus surgery. Otolaryngol Head Neck Surg 1994;110: 406–12.

55. Purkey MT, Smith TL, Ferguson BJ, et al. Subcutaneous immunotherapy for allergic rhinitis: an evidence based review of the recent literature with recommendations. Int Forum Allergy Rhinol 2013;3:519–31.

56. Loftus PA, Wise SK. Allergic fungal rhinosinusitis: the latest in diagnosis and management. Adv Otorhinolaryngol 2016;79:13–20.

57. Ferguson BJ, Barnes L, Bernstein JM, et al. Geographic variation in allergic fungal rhinosinusitis. Otolaryngol Clin North Am 2000;33:441–9.

58. Patadia MO, Welch KC. Role of immunotherapy in allergic fungal rhinosinusitis. Curr Opin Otolaryngol Head Neck Surg 2015;23:21–8.

59. Wise SK, Ghegan MD, Gorham E, et al. Socioeconomic factors in the diagnosis of allergic fungal rhinosinusitis. Otolaryngol Head Neck Surg 2008;138:38–42.

60. Wise SK, Venkatraman G, Wise JC, et al. Ethnic differences in bone erosion in allergic fungal sinusitis. Am J Rhinol 2004;18:397–404.

61. Lu-Myers Y, Deal AM, Miller JD, et al. Comparison of socioeconomic and demographic factors in patients with chronic rhinosinusitis and allergic fungal rhinosinusitis. Otolaryngol Head Neck Surg 2015;153:137–43.

62. Katzenstein AL, Sale SR, Greenberger PA. Allergic aspergillus sinusitis: a newly recognized form of sinusitis. J Allergy Clin Immunol 1983;72:89–93.

63. Manning SC, Schaefer SD, Close LG, et al. Culture-positive allergic fungal sinusitis. Arch Otolaryngol Head Neck Surg 1991;117:174–8.

64. Bent JP 3rd, Kuhn FA. Diagnosis of allergic fungal sinusitis. Otolaryngol Head Neck Surg 1994;111:580–8.

65. Lanza DC, Kennedy DW. Adult rhinosinusitis defined. Otolaryngol Head Neck Surg 1997;117:S1–7.

66. Plonk DP, Luong A. Current understanding of allergic fungal rhyinosinusitis and treatment implications. Curr Opin Otolaryngol Head Neck Surg 2014;22:221–6.

67. Callejas CA, Douglas RG. Fungal rhinosinusitis: what every allergist should know. Clin Exp Allergy 2013;43:835–49.

68. Silva MP, Baroody FM. Allergic fungal rhinosinusitis. Ann Allergy Asthma Immunol 2013;110:217–22.
69. Pant H, Kette FE, Smith WB, et al. Fungal-specific humoral response in eosinophilic mucus chronic rhinosinusitis. Laryngoscope 2005;115:601–6.
70. Saravanan K, Panda NK, Chakrabarti A, et al. Allergic fungal rhinosinusitis: an attempt to resolve the diagnostic dilemma. Arch Otolaryngol Head Neck Surg 2006;132:173–8.
71. Hutcheson PS, Schubert MS, Slavin RG. Distinctions between allergic fungal rhinosinusitis and chronic rhinosinusitis. Am J Rhinol Allergy 2010;24: 405–8.
72. Matsuwaki Y, Uno K, Okushi T, et al. Total and antigen-(fungi, mites, and staphylococcal enterotoxins) specific IgEs in nasal polyps is related to local eosinophilic inflammation. Int Arch Allergy Immunol 2013;161:147–53.
73. Chang YT, Fang SY. Tissue-specific immunoglobulin E in maxillary sinus mucosa of allergic fungal sinusitis. Rhinology 2008;46:226–30.
74. Wise SK, Ahn CN, Lathers DM, et al. Antigen-specific IgE in sinus mucosa of allergic fungal rhinosinusitis patients. Am J Rhinol 2008;22:451–6.
75. Collins M, Nair S, Smith W, et al. Role of local immunoglobulin E production in the pathophysiology of noninvasive fungal sinusitis. Laryngoscope 2004;114: 1242–6.
76. Ragab A, Samak RM. Immunohistochemical dissimilarity between allergic fungal and nonfungal chronic rhinosinusitis. Am J Rhinol Allergy 2013;27:168–76.
77. MacKenzie JR, Mattes J, Dent LA, et al. Eosinophils promote allergic disease of the lung by regulating CD4 Th2 lymphocyte function. J Immunol 2001;167: 3146–55.
78. Garro AP, Chiapello LS, Baronetti JL, et al. Rat eosinophils stimulate the expansion of Cryptococcus neoformans-specific CD4(+) and CD8(+) T cells with a T-helper 1 profile. Immunology 2011;132:174–87.
79. Bassichis BA, Marple BF, Mabry RL, et al. Use of immunotherapy in previously treated patients with allergic fungal sinusitis. Otolaryngol Head Neck Surg 2001;125:487–90.
80. Mabry RL, Marple BF, Mabry CS. Outcomes after discontinuing immunotherapy for allergic fungal sinusitis. Otolaryngol Head Neck Surg 2000;122:104–6.
81. Mabry RL, Mabry CS. Allergic fungal sinusitis: the role of immunotherapy. Otolaryngol Clin North Am 2000;33:433–40.
82. Mabry RL, Manning SC, Mabry CS. Immunotherapy for allergic fungal sinusitis. Otolaryngol Head Neck Surg 1997;116:31–5.
83. Mabry RL, Mabry CS. Immunotherapy for allergic fungal sinusitis: the second year. Otolaryngol Head Neck Surg 1997;117:367–71.
84. Mabry RL, Marple BF, Folker RJ, et al. Immunotherapy for allergic fungal sinusitis: three years' experience. Otolaryngol Head Neck Surg 1998;119:648–51.
85. Melzer JM, Driskill BR, Clenney TL, et al. Sublingual immunotherapy for allergic fungal sinusitis. Ann Otol Rhinol Laryngol 2015;124:782–7.
86. Gan EC, Habib AR, Rajwani A, et al. Omalizumab therapy for refractory allergic fungal rhinosinusitis patients with moderate or severe asthma. Am J Otolaryngol 2015;36:672–7.
87. Folker RJ, Marple BF, Mabry RL, et al. Treatment of allergic fungal sinusitis: a comparision trial of postoperative immunotherapy with specific fungal antigens. Laryngoscope 1998;108:1623–7.

88. Marple BF, Newcomer M, Schwade N, et al. Natural history of allergic fungal rhinosinusitis: a 4 to 10 year follow up. Otolaryngol Head Neck Surg 2002;127: 361–6.
89. deShazo RD, Swain RE. Diagnostic criteria for allergic fungal sinusitis. J Allergy Clin Immunol 1995;96:24–35.

The Role of Allergy in Otologic Disease

Betty Yang, MD, Christopher D. Brook, MD*

KEYWORDS

- Allergy • Atopy • Eustachian tube • Otitis media with effusion • Ménière's disease
- Endolymphatic hydrops • Eosinophilic otitis media • Immunotherapy

KEY POINTS

- The current medical evidence supports the relationship between allergic disease, eustachian tube dysfunction, and otitis media with effusion.
- Atopic disease may play a role in the pathogenesis of eosinophilic otitis media.
- The association of allergy and Ménière's disease is well-documented, and certain patients may benefit from allergy immunotherapy.

INTRODUCTION

Allergic disease is one of the most common conditions for which patients seek treatment in the United States. The prevalence of allergy has been estimated at around 30% to 40%,[1] and the economic burden of allergic rhinitis has been estimated to be between $5.5 and $9.7 billion per year.[2] Allergy is commonly associated with conditions such as rhinitis, sinusitis, and asthma, but the relationship between allergy and otologic disease is less clear. In this article, the authors examine the evidence for a relationship between allergic disease and several common otologic conditions, including otitis media, eosinophilic otitis media (EOM), and Ménière's disease (MD).

THE ROLE OF ALLERGY IN EUSTACHIAN TUBE DYSFUNCTION AND OTITIS MEDIA WITH EFFUSION

Otitis media with effusion (OME) is a clinical disease characterized by the presence of nonpurulent fluid in the middle ear behind an intact tympanic membrane. The symptoms of OME usually involve hearing loss and aural fullness; in children, it can be associated with delayed speech and language development and may cause permanent middle ear damage with mucosal changes.[3] Although it is generally agreed that

Disclosure Statement: The authors have no conflicts of interest to disclose.
Department of Otolaryngology–Head and Neck Surgery, Boston University Medical Center, 820 Harrison Avenue, FGH Building 4th Floor, Boston, MA 02118, USA
* Corresponding author.
E-mail address: cdbrook@gmail.com

OME is a multifactorial disease arising from various factors including viral or bacterial pathogens, environmental risks such as firsthand or secondhand smoking, and patient-specific anatomy, the relationship between allergy and OME has been historically controversial.

Epidemiology

Many recent studies have established that the prevalence of allergic rhinitis in patients with OME is higher than that in the general population, although the degree of difference in these studies varies greatly. In Korea, the incidence of allergic rhinitis was significantly higher in children with OME (33.8%) than without OME (16%).[4] In Japan, it was estimated that 6% to 20% of the general population is atopic and, among atopic patients, only 21% have OME; however, more than 87% of patients with OME were found to be atopic and/or have allergy symptoms.[5] In other studies, allergy is estimated to confer anywhere from a 2.0- to a 4.5-fold increased incidence of OME compared with that of nonsensitized people.[6,7] The wide range of prevalence may be attributed to uncontrolled study designs, including varying criteria used for diagnosing allergic sensitization and the different populations being studied.[8,9]

Pathophysiology

The accumulation of fluid in the middle ear cavity in OME involves 2 different mechanisms at the level of the middle ear mucosa: the first involves transduction from the mucosa capillaries, and the second involves active secretion, or exudation, from mucosal glands.[10] The eustachian tube (ET) also plays a role and is a structure that facilitates communication between the middle ear cavity with the nasopharynx. Its basic functions are (1) ventilating the middle ear cavity to regulate middle ear air pressure with atmospheric pressure, replenishing oxygen that has been absorbed and allowing gases produced in the middle ear to escape, (2) draining middle ear secretions into the nasopharynx, and (3) protecting the middle ear from nasopharyngeal secretions and sound pressure.[11] The respiratory epithelium lining the ET mucosa has several types of defense mechanisms, including mechanical (eg, mucociliary apparatus), innate (eg, inflammatory mediators), and acquired (eg, antigen specific).[12] It has been established that OME is related to ET dysfunction, because suboptimal opening and closing of the ET affects the basic functions of ventilating and draining the middle ear space.[9,13,14] The proposed mechanisms explain that ET dysfunction is due to an inflammatory process that includes intrinsic mechanical obstruction from the inflammatory swelling of the ET mucosa, altered mucociliary activity, and hypersecretion by seromucous glands. Several double-blind protocols have demonstrated intranasal allergen challenges result in ET obstruction, with allergic reaction inhibiting even transient dilations of the ET during swallowing.[15–18] Histologic studies have also shown that levels of eosinophils, CD3 T cells, interleukin (IL)-4 levels, and messenger RNA levels for IL-5 are increased at both ends of the ET. All these studies suggest that the ET may become dysfunctional owing to allergic inflammation causing intrinsic mucosal edema and obstruction.

The adenoidal tissues are part of the mucosal-associated lymphoid tissue of the upper airway as well, joining the palatine, torus tubarius, and lingual tonsils to form the circle of lymphoid tissue around the pharyngeal wall known as Waldeyer's ring. The adenoids are organized in deep crypts, and contain germinal centers and interfollicular areas, which play an important role in the generation of both T helper cells (Th1, Th2), and immunoglobulin A (IgA)-committed B cells.[19] Adenoids have been proposed to cause ET dysfunction both by physical obstruction as well as by the release of chemical mediators. The proportions of $CD4^+$, $CD8^+$, and $CD19^+$ associated with Bcl-2 (an antiapoptotic protein) were found to be lower in children with hypertrophic adenoids with OME than the levels in children with hypertrophic adenoids without OME, which indicates there is enhanced apoptosis of the naïve and effector T cells in adenoid tissue, suggesting the adenoids play a role in lymphocyte regulation in local immunologic disorders.[20] Another study reported that lymphocytes from the adenoids showed decreased Th1 cytokine but normal Th2 cytokine secretions compared with peripheral blood lymphocytes among children with recurrent otitis media, which suggests the underlying Th2 immune profile associated with atopy may play a role in determining the risk of recurrent OME.[21]

The middle ear mucosa evolves from the same ectoderm as the rest of the upper respiratory tract epithelium, and has been found in animal studies to have the same active intrinsic immunologic responsiveness to antigenic stimulus as the nasal tract, sinuses, and bronchi.[22] Inflammatory cells and molecules found in the fluid of middle ear effusions (MEEs) have been used to evaluate the pathogenesis of OME. Several studies have reported increased eosinophil mediators and increased Th2 cytokine levels in MEEs and mucosal biopsies.[23–27] One such study in adults revealed that levels of IL-4 were higher in MEEs of adults with allergic rhinitis than in those without allergic rhinitis, suggesting that Th2 cytokines may be related to the pathogenesis of OME in allergic rhinitis–positive adults, whereas Th1 cytokines potentially affect MEEs in OME regardless of the presence of allergic rhinitis.[28] Multiple other studies have demonstrated the association of serum and middle ear immunoglobulins with Th2 response in the middle ear.[29–31] These studies suggest that inflammation of the middle ear can indeed be allergic in nature, and the middle ear may be included with the rest of the upper respiratory tract in the concept of the single "unified airway."[29,32]

Immunotherapy for Otitis Media with Effusion

There are studies investigating immunotherapy and OME that have demonstrated that some patients' effusions resolve when allergies are treated with immunotherapy and/or diet elimination, although these trials are uncontrolled or nonrandomized.[33–40] In 2008, Hurst[41] conducted a study comparing immunotherapy treatment patients with a control cohort of allergic patients not receiving immunotherapy, showing resolution of 89% of OME in treated patients versus 0% of controls. This study suggested that, in this select population, immunotherapy was efficacious in preventing or limiting the duration of OME; however, this study was not randomized, and a possibility of a strong selection bias exists without randomization, limiting the ability to come to a scientific conclusion based on these data alone.[41]

Summary

The current medical evidence supports the relationship between allergic disease, ET dysfunction, and OME. The majority of studies that have been performed on this subject suggest that a large percentage of patients with OME are atopic, and that the middle ear is capable of an allergic response and can be considered a part of the unified airway. Definitive randomized studies on resolution of effusions with immunotherapy are lacking, and future randomized, controlled trials are needed to determine the exact role of allergen immunotherapy in the OME population.

EOSINOPHILIC OTITIS MEDIA

EOM is a form of intractable otitis media that occurs primarily in patients with bronchial asthma and was first reported in 1994.[42] The diagnostic criteria for EOM were established in 2011, and since then the pathophysiology and clinical characteristics of the disease are continuing to be elucidated.[43–47] The major criteria are identification of eosinophils from MEE or middle ear mucosa by histologic or cytologic examination. Minor diagnostic criteria include association with adult-onset bronchial asthma and nasal polyposis, highly viscous MEE, and resistance to conventional treatment for otitis media. A definitive case meets the major criteria plus 2 or more minor criteria.[43]

Epidemiology

The majority of first-time EOM patients have been found to be aged 50 to 60 years, with a 2:1 female to male ratio.[43] On average, these patients showed an 83% rate of bilateral disease a 50% rate of superimposed progressive sensorineural hearing loss, and a 6% rate of hearing loss progression to complete deafness in the involved ears.[43] Approximately 75% displayed sinusitis or multiple nasal polyps and adult-onset bronchial asthma.[43]

Clinical Features

EOM is generally considered to be a bilateral process. Regardless of the existence of tympanic membrane perforation, the effusion of EOM is yellowish and highly viscous. When a tympanostomy tube is placed in EOM, the lumen of the tube is easily blocked by the viscous effusion.[48] In a study of 190 EOM patients, approximately one-half showed conductive hearing loss and 6% became completely deaf.[43] It is proposed that eosinophilic and bacterial inflammatory products of the middle ear may invade the inner ear via the round window to cause inner ear damage.[48] Risk factors associated with the severity of EOM include body mass index and duration of bronchial asthma.[49] The prevalence of eosinophilic rhinosinusitis has been found to be increased in patients with EOM at approximately 75%,[48] another disease often associated with an atopic Th2 inflammatory pattern.

Pathophysiology

ET dysfunction, specifically insufficient closing of the ET as evaluated by sonotubometry, has been observed in EOM patients and may lead to pathogenic EOM by allowing foreign materials to enter the middle ear and cause eosinophilic inflammation.[50,51] Histologic examination of the MEEs in EOM patients have shown the level of IgE as well as the concentration of eosinophil cationic protein are significantly higher in the MEE than the serum of EOM patients.[52] Eosinophilic granule 2–positive cells and the eosinophil chemoattractants IL-5 and eotaxin have been found to be significantly higher in the MEE and middle ear mucosa of EOM patients than in the corresponding control group.[53,54] Another study examined a population of 26 patients with EOM and found that there were a high number of positive sensitizations in serum testing (16 of 26 had positive testing to perennial allergens), and that the rate of detection of specific IgE locally within the ear was significantly higher than in control patients. They found that antigen-specific IgE within the middle ear was present in 16 of 26 patients versus 1 of 9 control patients ($P \leq .01$), and that middle ear–specific IgE presence correlated with the severity of EOM, suggesting a role for atopic disease in the pathogenesis of EOM and perhaps presenting a therapeutic target.[55]

Treatment

Standard treatment for EOM differs around the world. In some places, steroids are injected into the middle ears, and supplanted with antibiotics as indicated by infection. The anti-IgE agent omalizumab has also been shown to improve the severity of EOM with resolution of MEE; however, the clinical application of omalizumab may be limited by its cost and need for prolonged use.[49,56] A recent study showed promise in weekly injections of pegylated interferon in the treatment of refractory cases of EOM.[51]

In the United States, EOM treatment still seems to focus on surgical intervention. Surgical treatment with tympanostomy tubes as mentioned does not effectively solve the clinical symptoms of EOM. Tympanoplasty is aimed at controlling otorrhea or treating hearing impairment owing to EOM, and tympanomastoidectomy facilitates middle ear and mastoid ventilation, and the delivery of topical steroids. There have also been cases reported in which cochlear implantation was performed to treat deafness associated with EOM.[57,58]

Future study will be needed to determine the role for allergy treatment and immunotherapy in this challenging disease. It stands to reason that, a Th2-driven disease with high levels of local specific IgE, may benefit from immunotherapy, but at this time the question remains unanswered.

Summary

EOM is a recently described entity, the pathophysiology of which seems to be related to chronic allergic or immune response, likely through antigen presentation via a dysfunctional ET. The clinical features of this disease are still being defined through case reports and series, and further research is needed in identifying the role of allergy in the pathophysiology and treatment.

ALLERGY AND ENDOLYMPHATIC HYDROPS

The symptoms of MD were first described by Prosper Ménière in 1861, when he associated episodes of vertigo with the inner ear. The syndrome is described by the American Academy of Otolaryngology-Head and Neck Surgery (AAO-HNS) as the presence of recurrent, spontaneous episodic vertigo (rotational and lasting at least 20 minutes), hearing loss, aural fullness, and tinnitus (**Table 1**).[59] It is generally agreed that the pathogenesis of MD involves the hydropic distension of the endolymphatic system, and the AAO-HNS also describes MD as the "idiopathic syndrome of endolymphatic

Table 1 Criteria for diagnosis of Ménière's disease	
Diagnostic Certainty	**Criteria**
Certain	Definite Ménière's disease, plus histopathologic confirmation of hydrops
Definite	Two or more spontaneous episodes of vertigo, each lasting 20 min to 12 h Audiometrically documented low-frequency to midfrequency sensorineural hearing loss in 1 ear, defining the affected ear on at least 1 occasion before, during, or after 1 of the episodes of vertigo Fluctuating aural symptoms (hearing, tinnitus, or fullness) in the affected ear not better accounted for by another vestibular diagnosis
Probable	Two or more episodes of vertigo or dizziness, each lasting 20 min to 24 h; fluctuating aural symptoms (hearing, tinnitus, or fullness) in the affected ear not better accounted for by another vestibular diagnosis
Possible	Episodic vertigo of the Ménière's type without documented hearing loss or sensorineural hearing loss, fluctuating or fixed, with disequilibrium but without definite episodes Other causes excluded

hydrops." Although by definition idiopathic, MD has previously been attributed to a variety of etiologies including trauma, viral infections, metabolic disorders, autoimmune factors, and allergies. Although there is not yet any evidence to prove causation between allergy and MD, there has been a recognized association between the 2 entities for nearly a century; the first published report of MD thought to be related to allergy appeared in the literature in 1923, when 2 cases were described of patients with symptoms consistent with MD whose symptoms resolved with epinephrine treatment.[60] An association between allergy and MD has been shown in various cross-sectional and observational studies over time.

Epidemiology

In the United States, MD has been reported as having an incidence rate of 15 per 100,000 and a prevalence rate of 190 per 100,000.[61,62] The prevalence in Japan and Finland have been reported as 17 per 100,000 and 43 per 100,000, respectively.[63] In a survey of 734 patients with Ménière's syndrome, the prevalence of skin test–confirmed concurrent allergic disease was 41%, roughly 3 times the prevalence of physician-diagnosed allergy in the general population.[64,65]

Pathophysiology

The exact pathophysiology of MD is poorly understood, although it is generally believed to be related to distortion of the membranous labyrinth resulting from an overaccumulation of endolymph. The inner ear fluids endolymph and perilymph are separated by thin membranes that support the neural apparatus of hearing and balance. Attacks of hydrops are proposed to be due to an increase in endolymphatic pressure, which causes a rupture in Reissner's membrane separating the perilymph from endolymph. The resulting chemical mixture leads to depolarization blockade and transient loss of function of the vestibular nerve. This sudden change in the firing rate of the vestibular nerve creates an acute vestibular imbalance, or vertigo.[66]

It has been suggested that the endolymphatic sac and duct are the sites of immune activity in the inner ear. The endolymphatic sac has been found to be capable of both processing antigens and producing its own local antibody response.[67,68] IgG, IgM, IgA, and secretory components are found in the endolymphatic sac, and the perisaccular connective tissue houses numerous plasma cells, macrophages, as well as mast cells.[69,70]

A few mechanisms by which allergy could produce MD have been proposed, with a focus on the theme of inflammation within the endolymphatic sac[71] are as follows:

1. The endolymphatic sac contains fenestrated blood vessels that allow for antigen entry, subsequently leading to mast cell degranulation and inflammation in the perisaccular connective tissue. This could then result in a toxic accumulation of metabolic products, which may interfere with hair cell function, and the histamine release could cause vasodilation and affect the resorptive capacity of the endolymphatic sac.
2. Circulating immune complexes enter the endolymphatic sac circulation through the fenestrated blood vessels or are deposited in the stria, resulting in inflammation and possibly increased vascular permeability, disrupting the normal fluid balance in the inner ear.
3. A viral antigen–allergic interaction stimulates Waldeyer's ring, triggering T-cell migration to the endolymphatic sac, which results in a chronic low-grade inflammation and, over time, can stimulate excess fluid production.

Treatment

The aim of medical treatment of MD is symptomatic relief. The standard therapy for MD involves a sodium-restricted diet, diuretic medication, and vestibulosuppressants as needed, which for the majority of patients offers acceptable relief from vertigo. No treatment has been found thus far for stabilization of the hearing loss resulting from MD. In MD that has failed medical therapy, further interventions can be trialed including use of a Meniette pressure-regulating device, intratympanic gentamicin, endolymphatic shunt surgery, or ablative procedures such as vestibular nerve section or labyrinthectomy.[71,72]

Betahistine is a medication commonly prescribed for the treatment of MD. It is a histamine analogue medication that acts as a weak H1 receptor agonist and strong H3 receptor antagonist. Its proposed mechanism is decreasing the release of histamine, dopamine, gamma-aminobutyric acid, acetylcholine, norepinephrine, and serotonin, improving microcirculation in the inner ear.[73] Although it is one of the most frequently prescribed medications for MD in Europe, it is not currently available in the United States, although can be obtained by compounding pharmacies or through sources in Canada or Europe.[74,75] Prior observational studies and randomized, controlled trials produced contradictory results on the treatment efficacy of betahistine; however, a recent large double-blind randomized placebo controlled trial provided no clear evidence that betahistine produces a significant decrease in the number of vertigo attacks.[76]

The most commonly prescribed medications for the treatment of MD in the United States are antihistamines, including meclizine, diphenhydramine, and dimenhydrinate. It is thought that these medications exert an anticholinergic central suppressive effect on vertigo. These medications ultimately do not alter the underlying pathology of hydropic distention of the endolymphatic space.

The effect of allergen immunotherapy and elimination of suspected food allergens in MD patients has been studied. There was a significant improvement from before to after treatment in both allergy and MD symptoms in those treated with allergen immunotherapy and dietary avoidance in one retrospective study.[77] A subsequent prospective questionnaire-based study demonstrated a significant decrease of vertigo, tinnitus, and unsteadiness, and improvement of ratings on AAO-HNS disability scale after immunotherapy, suggesting a role for allergen immunotherapy in this disease.[71]

Summary

Although MD is accepted to be a multifactorial disease, the association of allergy and MD is well-documented, and allergy may be involved in the final inflammatory pathway in certain patients with MD.[78] The research on MD and allergy treatment is largely made up of clinical case reports, with a lack of any randomized, double-blind, placebo-controlled trials comparing MD patient outcomes with immunotherapy; however, it is suggested that immunotherapy and dietary avoidance of allergens do lessen the severity of MD symptoms. The available evidence is in the form of prospective cohort studies, which suggest possible symptomatic improvement with allergy immunotherapy. These suppositions are made with uncontrolled studies, and one must take into consideration that MD often has a fluctuating course with periods of quiescence. Continued research is needed to more definitively demonstrate the benefits of these treatments; however, in the right patients, the risk of immunotherapy and dietary avoidance is low and can be considered in patients with MD who demonstrate allergic symptoms or have positive allergy testing.

REFERENCES

1. American College of Asthma, Allergy and Immunology. Allergy facts. Available at: http://www.acaai.org/news/facts-statistics/allergies. Accessed April 29, 2017.
2. Reed SD, Lee TA, McCrory DC. The economic burden of allergic rhinitis: a critical evaluation of the literature. Pharmacoeconomics 2004;22:345–61.
3. Teele DW, Klein JO, Rosner B. Otitis media with effusion during the first three years of life and the development of speech and language. Pediatrics 1984;74: 282–6.
4. Kwon C, Lee HY, Kim GM, et al. Allergic diseases in children with otitis media with effusion. Int J Pediatr Otorhinolaryngol 2013;77:158–61.
5. Tomonaga K, Kurono Y, Moge G. The role of nasal allergy in otitis media with effusion, a clinical study. Acta Otolaryngol Suppl 1988;458:41–7.
6. Stenstrom C, Ingvarsson L. General illness and need of medical care in otitis prone children. Int J Pediatr Otorhinolaryngol 1994;29(1):23–32.
7. Chantzi FM, Kafetzis DA, Bairamis T, et al. IgE sensitization, respiratory allergy symptoms, and heritability independently increase the risk of otitis media with effusion. Allergy 2006;61(3):332–6.
8. Miccli Sopo S, Zorzi G, Calvani M Jr. Should we screen every child with otitis media with effusion for allergic rhinitis? Arch Dis Child 2004;89(3):287–8.
9. Tewfik TL, Mazer B. The links between allergy and otitis media with effusion. Curr Opin Otolaryngol Head Neck Surg 2006;14(3):187–90.
10. Oh J, Kim WJ. Interaction between allergy and middle ear infection. Curr Allergy Asthma Rep 2016;16:66.
11. Bernstein JM. Role of allergy in eustachian tube blockage and otitis media with effusion: a review. Otolaryngol Head Neck Surg 1996;114(4):562–8.
12. Murphy TF, Chonmaitree T, Barenkamp S, et al. Panel 5: microbiology and immunology panel. Otolaryngol Head Neck Surg 2013;148(4 Suppl):E64–89.
13. Fireman P. Otitis media and eustachian tube dysfunction: connection to allergic rhinitis. J Allergy Clin Immunol 1997;99(2):787–97.
14. Pelikan Z. The role of nasal allergy in chronic secretory otitis media. Ann Allergy Asthma Immunol 2007;99(5):401–7.
15. Ackerman M, Friedman R, Doyle W, et al. Antigen-induced eustachian tube obstruction: an internasal provocative challenge test. J Allergy Clin Immunol 1984;73:604–9.
16. Skoner DP, Doyle WJ, Chamovitz AH, et al. Eustachian tube obstruction after internasal challenge with house dust mite. Arch Otolaryngol Head Neck Surg 1986; 112:840–2.
17. Friedman RA, Doyle WJ, Casselbrant ML, et al. Immunologic-mediated eustachian tube obstruction: a double-blind crossover study. J Allergy Clin Immunol 1983;71:442–7.
18. Doyle WE, Takahara T, Fireman P. The role of allergy in the pathogenesis of otitis media with effusion. Arch Otolaryngol 1985;111:502–6.
19. Van Kempen MJ, Rijkers GT, Van Cauwenberge PB. The immune response in adenoids and tonsils. Int Arch Allergy Immunol 2000;122(1):8–19.
20. Zelazowska-Rutkowska B, Wysocka J, Skotnicka B. Chosen factors of T and B cell apoptosis in hypertrophic adenoid in children with otitis media with effusion. Int J Pediatr Otorhinolaryngol 2010;74(6):698–700.
21. Bernstein JM, Ballow M, Xiang S, et al. Th1/Th2 cytokine profiles in the nasopharyngeal lymphoid tissues of children with recurrent otitis media. Ann Otol Rhinol Laryngol 1998;107(1):22–7.

22. Takeuchi K, Tomemori T, Iriyoshi N, et al. Analysis of T cell receptor b chain reper-toire in middle ear effusions. Ann Otol Rhinol Laryngol 1996;105:213–7.

23. Hurst DS. Association of otitis media with effusion and allergy as demonstrated by intradermal skin testing and eosinophil cationic protein levels in both middle ear effusions and mucosal biopsies. Laryngoscope 1996;106(9):1128–37.

24. Hurst DS, Venge P. Evidence of eosinophil, neutrophil, and mast-cell mediators in the effusion of OME patients with and without atopy. Allergy 2000;55(5):435–41.

25. Jang CH, Kim YH. Characterization of cytokines present in pediatric otitis media without effusion: comparison of allergy positive and negative. Int J Pediatr Otorhi-nolaryngol 2002;66:37–40.

26. Hotomi M, Samukawa T, Yamanoka N. Interleukin-B in otitis media with effusion. Acta Otolaryngol 1994;114:406–9.

27. Wright ED, Hurst D, Miono D, et al. Increased expression of major basic protein (MBP) and interleukin-5 (IL-5) in middle ear biopsy specimens from atopic pa-tients with persistent otitis media with effusion. Otolaryngol Head Neck Surg 2000;123:533–8.

28. Kariya S, Okano M, Hattori H, et al. TH1/TH2 and regulatory cytokines in adults with otitis media with effusion. Otol Neurotol 2006;27:1089–93.

29. Nguyen LH, Manoukian JJ, Sobol SB, et al. Similar allergic inflammation in the middle ear and the upper airway: evidence linking otitis media with effusion to the unified airway concept. J Allergy Clin Immunol 2004;114:1110–5.

30. Lasisi AO, Arinola OG, Olayemi O. Role of elevated immunoglobuline E levels in suppurative otitis media. Ann Trop Paediatr 2008;28:123–7.

31. Hurst DS, Weakley M, Yamanarayaman MP. Evidence of possible localized spe-cific immunoglobulin E production in middle ear fluid as demonstrated by ELISA testing. Otolaryngol Head Neck Surg 1999;121:224–30.

32. Braunstahl GJ, Overbeek SE, Kleinjan A, et al. Nasal allergen provocation in-duces adhesion molecule expression and tissue eosinophilia in upper and lower airways. J Allergy Clin Immunol 2001;107(3):469–76.

33. Jordan R. Chronic secretory otitis media. Laryngoscope 1949;59(9):1002–15.

34. Whitcomb NJ. Allergy therapy in serous otitis media associated with allergic rhinitis. Ann Allergy 1965;23:232–6.

35. Draper WL. Secretory otitis media in children: a study of 540 children. Laryngo-scope 1967;77:636–53.

36. Hall LJ, Lukat RM. Results of allergy treatment on the Eustachian tube in chronic serous otitis media. Am J Otol 1981;3(2):116–21.

37. McMahan JT, Calenoff E, Croft DJ, et al. Chronic otitis media with effusion and allergy: modified RAST analysis of 119 cases. Otolaryngol Head Neck Surg 1981;89(3 Pt 1):427–31.

38. Hurst DS. Allergy management of refractory serous otitis media. Otolaryngol Head Neck Surg 1990;102(6):664–9.

39. Nsouli TM, Nsouli SM, Linde RE, et al. The role of food allergy in serous otitis me-dia. Ann Allergy 1994;73(3):215.

40. Psifidis A, Hatzistilianou M, Samaras K, et al. Atopy and otitis media inn children. Paper presented at Proceedings of the 7th International Congress of Pediatric Otorhinolaryngology. Helsinki, Finland, July 8-10, 1998.

41. Hurst DS. Efficacy of allergy immunotherapy as a treatment for patients with chronic otitis media with effusion. Int J Pediatr Otorhinolaryngol 2008;72(8): 1215–23.

42. Tomioka S, Kobayashi T, Takasaka T, et al. Intractable otitis media in patients with bronchial asthma (eosinophilic otitis media). In: Sanna M, editor. Cholesteatoma and mastoid surgery. Rome (Italy): CIC Edizioni Internazionali; 1997. p. 851–3.

43. Iino Y, Tomioka-Matsutani S, Matsubara A, et al. Diagnostic criteria of eosinophilic otitis media, a newly recognized middle ear disease. Auris Nasus Larynx 2011; 38(4):456–61.

44. Childers AL, Gruen J, Sayeed S, et al. Eosinophilic otitis media. Otol Neurotol 2014;35:206–7.

45. Chung WJ, Lee JH, Lim HK, et al. Eosinophilic otitis media: CT and MRI findings and literature review. Korean J Radiol 2012;13:363–7.

46. Turkmen MT, Yagiz R. A case of intractable otitis media: eosinophilic otitis media. Balkan Med J 2014;31(3):268–9.

47. Vazquez A, Blake DM, Jyung RW. Eosinophilic otitis media. Ear Nose Throat J 2014;93:27.

48. Kanazawa H, Yoshida N, Iino Y. New insights into eosinophilic otitis media. Curr Allergy Asthma Rep 2015;15:76.

49. Iino Y, Hara M, Hasegawa M, et al. Clinical efficacy of anti-IgE therapy for eosinophilic otitis media. Otol Neurotol 2012;33:1218–24.

50. Iino Y, Kakizaki K, Saruya S, et al. Eustachian tube function in patients with eosinophilic otitis media associated with bronchial asthma evaluated by sonotubometry. Arch Otolaryngol Head Neck Surg 2006;132:1109–14.

51. Neff BA, Voss SG, Carlson ML, et al. Treatment of eosinophilic otitis media with pegylated interferon-α 2a and 2b. Laryngoscope 2017;127:1208–16.

52. Iino Y. Role of IgE in eosinophilic otitis media. Allergol Int 2010;59:233–8.

53. Nonaka M, Fukumoto A, Ozu C, et al. I-5 and eotaxin levels in middle ear effusion and blood from asthmatics with otitis media with effusion. Acta Otolaryngol 2003; 123:383–7.

54. Iino Y, Kakizaki K, Katano H, et al. Eosinophil chemoattractant in middle ear patients with eosinophilic otitis media. Clin Exp Allergy 2005;35:1370–6.

55. Kanazawa H, Yoshida N, Shinnabe A, et al. Antigen-specific IgE in middle ear effusion of patients with eosinophilic otitis media. Ann Allergy Asthma Immunol 2014;113(1):88–92.

56. Okude A, Tagaya E, Kondo M, et al. A case of severe asthma with eosinophilic otitis media successfully treated with anti-IgE monoclonal antibody omalizumab. Case Rep Pulmonol 2012;2012:340525.

57. Iwasaki S, Nagura M, Mizuta K. Cochlear implantation in a patient with eosinophilic otitis media. Eur Arch Otorhinolaryngol 2006;263:365–9.

58. Kojima H, Sakurai Y, Rikitake M, et al. Cochlear implantation in patients with chronic otitis media. Auris Nasus Larynx 2010;37:415–21.

59. American Academy of Otolaryngology – Head and Neck Foundation. Committee on hearing and equilibrium guidelines for the diagnosis and evaluation of therapy in Ménière's disease. Otolaryngol Head Neck Surg 1995;113:181–5.

60. Duke WW. Ménière's Syndrome caused by allergy. JAMA 1923;81(26):2179–81.

61. Wladislavosky-Wasserman P, Facer GW, Mokri B, et al. Ménière's disease: a 30-year epidemiologic and clinical study in Rochester, MN, 1951-1980. Laryngoscope 1984;94:1098–102.

62. Harris JP, Alexander TH. Current-day prevalence of Ménière's syndrome. Audiol Neurootol 2010;15:318–22.

63. Sajjadi H, Paprella MM. Meniere's disease. Lancet 2008;372(9636):406–14.

64. Derebery MJ, Berliner KI. Prevalence of allergy in Ménière's disease. Otolaryngol Head Neck Surg 2000;123:69–75.

65. Allergies in America. A landmark survey of nasal allergy sufferers. Available at: http://www.myallergiesinamerica.com/. Accessed April 23, 2017.
66. Li JC, Lorenzo N, Egan RA, et al. Ménière disease (idiopathic endolymphatic hydrops). 2016. Available at: http://emedicine.medscape.com/article/1159069-overview?src=refgatesrc1#a4. Accessed April 24, 2017.
67. Harris JP. Immunology of the inner ear: evidence of local antibody production. Ann Otol Rhinol Laryngol 1984;93:157–62.
68. Tomiyama S, Harris JP. The role of the endolymphatic sac in inner ear immunity. Acta Otolaryngol 1987;103:182–8.
69. Altermatt HJ, Gebbers JO, Muller C, et al. Human endolymphatic sac: evidence for a role in inner ear immune defence. ORL J Otorhinolaryngol Relat Spec 1990; 52:143–8.
70. Uno K, Miyamura K, Kanzaki Y, et al. Type I allergy in the inner ear of the guinea pig. Ann Otol Rhinol Laryngol 1992;101(Suppl 157):78–81.
71. Derebery JM, Berliner KI. Allergy and its relation to Meniere's disease. Otolaryngol Clin North Am 2010;43:1047–58.
72. Dornhoffer JL, Kind D. The effect of the Meniett device in patients with Meniere's disease: long-term results. Otol Neurotol 2008;6:868–74.
73. Dagli M, Goksu N, Erylimaz A, et al. Expression of histamine receptors (H1, H2, and H3) in the rabbit endolymphatic sac: an immunohistochemical study. Am J Otolaryngol 2008;29:20–3.
74. Harcourt J, Barraclough K, Bronstein AM. Ménière's disease. BMJ 2014;349: g654.
75. Smith WK, Sankar V, Pfleiderer AG. A national survey amongst UK otolaryngologists regarding the treatment of Ménière's disease. J Laryngol Otol 2005;119: 102–5.
76. Adrion C, Fischer CS, Wagner J, et al. Efficacy and safety of betahistine treatment in patients with Ménière's disease: primary results of a long term, multicenter, double blind, randomized, placebo controlled, dose defining trial (BEMED trial). BMJ 2016;352:h6816.
77. Derebery MJ. Allergic management of Ménière's disease: an outcome study. Otolaryngol Head Neck Surg 2000;122:174–82.
78. Banks C, McGinness S, Harvey R, et al. Is allergy related to Ménière's disease? Curr Allergy Asthma Rep 2012;12:255–60.

Rational Approach to Allergy Testing

 CrossMark

Michael P. Platt, MD, MSc*, Jacqueline A. Wulu, MD

KEYWORDS

- Allergy testing • In vitro testing • Skin testing • Skin prick • Intradermal
- Allergic sensitization

KEY POINTS

- Identification of allergens for patients with allergic rhinitis is useful for confirmation of diagnosis, institution of avoidance measures, and formulation of immunotherapy plans.
- The clinical history is essential in the decision for allergy testing, method of testing, and interpretation of the results.
- Allergy testing can be performed by in vivo or in vitro methods. There are benefits and limitations to both methods, and the clinical scenario should determine the appropriate test for each patient.

INTRODUCTION

There is an increasing incidence of allergic diseases with up to 1 in 6 people affected by allergic rhinitis in the United States.[1] For patients with refractory symptoms of allergic rhinitis, allergy testing for identification of sensitizations is clinically useful for confirming the diagnosis, institution of avoidance measures, and formation of a desensitization protocol for immunotherapy. The decision to pursue allergy testing is based on clinical factors that include symptom severity, response to medical treatments, and potential usefulness of the positive test results. When deciding to pursue testing, there should be an identified benefit to understanding a patient's sensitizations. If the causative allergen is clear by history and there is no option of changing the environment or lack of interest in pursuing desensitization, testing may not be indicated. The clinical scenario is essential in determining the appropriateness of testing and type of test performed.

The diagnosis of allergic rhinitis remains a clinical entity in which history and physical examination with positive testing in appropriate circumstances are used for diagnosis. The history is essential in making the diagnosis of allergic rhinitis, deciding the

Disclosures: None.
Department of Otolaryngology–Head and Neck Surgery, Boston University School of Medicine, 820 Harrison Avenue, FGH Building, Boston, MA 02118, USA
* Corresponding author.
E-mail address: Miplatt@bu.edu

appropriate allergy tests, and interpreting the significance of positive test results. The information provided by the history regarding symptom quality and timing of symptoms in relation to season, exposures, and environments can often guide the physician to the classes of possible allergens. Because no allergy testing method is 100% sensitive or 100% specific, the clinical information is needed to apply the result of any allergy test to the clinical treatment plan.

A wide range of antigens can cause allergic reactions resulting in testing panels that can be unfeasibly large. Screening tests were created as a more effective means to determine the likelihood of someone having a particular allergic sensitization.[2] Screening tests often consist of antigens that the individual has previously encountered and are common in the geographic region. A representative of each allergen class with consideration of cross-reactivities within classes are used to formulate a screening panel. Screening tests typically contain 8 to 12 common environmental allergens that are typical for a particular geographic location or specific environmental exposure.[2]

Once the decision for testing has been made, the method of testing is dictated by factors in the clinical history and an informed decision by the patient. Because there is no perfect testing method, understanding what each test is measuring is important. Allergic rhinitis is an IgE-mediated disease in which IgE on mast cells leads to activation by binding of allergens and subsequent release of mediators such as histamine.[3] Commonly used tests for allergic rhinitis rely on either measurement of in vitro–specific binding of allergens to circulating IgE in the serum or the in vivo release of histamine by mast cells, which react with antigens placed in the skin.

In vitro testing measures circulating IgE, which comprises only a small percentage of the total IgE in the body. Most IgE is bound to mast cells within tissue; thus, testing of sera may fail to identify an existing sensitization (false-negative, lower sensitivity). Conversely, in vivo testing measures a skin reaction to an applied allergen, which may react positively because of a non–IgE-mediated trigger or alternate mechanism than by the intended antigen (false-positive, lower specificity). The presence of circulating IgE or skin reaction to allergens can only confirm the diagnosis of allergic rhinitis if the history and physical examination findings correlate with the test results. Direct nasal responses with nasal challenge tests are not typically used in clinical practice because of logistics, side effects, and risks of severe reactions.

Both in vivo and in vitro methods have benefits and limitations that are important to consider in clinical practice. When allergy tests results are positive despite lack of clinical symptoms, false-positive results must be considered. Alternately, negative results in the scenario of clinically reproducible symptoms at the time of exposure suggest possible false-negative results. The decision for method of testing and interpretation of results continues to be a clinical entity that relies on the history, physical examination, and interpretation of allergy testing results to determine the optimal treatment regimens for patients.

SKIN TESTING

In vivo skin testing evaluates the body's natural response to direct contact with an allergen. Skin testing was first described in 1872 when Dr Charles Blackley applied grass pollen to an abraded area of skin, causing an allergic response.[2] von Pirquet later performed skin testing for tuberculosis, prompting further development of skin testing. The scratch test was the first type of allergy skin test used, which consisted of applying the allergen into a scratched area on the forearm. Scratch testing is no longer performed secondary to inconsistent results, pain, and the risk of changes in skin pigmentation.[4,5]

Commonly used in vivo testing modalities include skin prick or puncture and intradermal testing. These skin tests use a small amount of antigen applied to the epidermis, commonly on the flexor aspect of the forearm or back while monitoring for an allergic response to both antigens and controls[6,7] which are typically read after 15 to 20 minutes.[4]

The prick or puncture method was developed in the 1950s by Sir Thomas Lewis.[6] The test consists of puncturing the epidermis either on the back or forearm allowing the allergen to penetrate the skin.[6] Positive and negative controls are placed at the time of testing samples, and both pediatric and adult patients maintain reliability in testing. This method of testing is often sought given the ease of performing the test and its lower risk of associated side effects compared with intradermal testing.[7]

Intradermal testing uses a small needle and syringe to inject a small volume of antigen into the dermis. An increased sensitivity is seen compared with skin prick testing, but there is also more discomfort, higher chance of allergic reaction, and an increased incidence of false-positive results because of the higher concentrations of exposure of antigen to the immune system.

Comparing intradermal testing with the prick method, intradermal testing has higher sensitivity. Negative results via the prick method can thus be corroborated by intradermal testing when there is clinical suspicion of a false-negative result. Additionally, for patients who are starting injection immunotherapy, the wheal size from the skin prick testing does not correlate as well as intradermal testing for selection of the starting dose for immunotherapy.[7,8] Peltier and Ryan[7] found that a positive wheal size of 4 to 6 mm would lead to initiating immunotherapy as 1, 2, and 3 dilutions more concentrated than the recommended starting point as determined by intradermal testing.[7]

There are other methods for gaining additional information regarding an individual's sensitivity level to an antigen. The intradermal dilutional method has a high specificity and provides quantitative values; however, this test is more invasive and costly and can lead to more discomfort for the patient.[7] The quantitative data are beneficial because this information can be used to estimate the initial dose of immunotherapy to be used.[5] Intradermal-guided immunotherapy can be initiated at higher concentrations and allows for quick up-titration even when the individual has a high antigen exposure secondary to the season.[7]

The modified quantitative testing (MQT) method uses both intradermal and skin prick techniques to gain the clinical information of sensitivity without the burdens of the intradermal dilutional method.[9] The MQT method starts with a skin prick response that then determines the concentration of intradermal test that is applied. This technique provides additional quantitative information about an individual's sensitivity and has been recognized as a valid form of testing by the American Academy of Otolaryngic Allergy.[2,7] Although MQT can take up to 45 minutes to perform, it is safe and effective in determining the initial dose when planning immunotherapy.[7]

There are clinical factors that limit the option for skin testing. Patients with diffuse dermatologic diseases such as dermatographism or severe eczema cannot be skin tested. Patients who are unable to stop medications that block histamine release will not have skin reactions to allergens or controls. Other contraindications include patients who take medication that interfere with treatment of anaphylaxis and pregnancy and highly sensitive patients who have a greater risk for severe systemic reaction or anaphylaxis. There are various factors that impact the results of in vivo testing such as medications, hormones, location of test site, and age.[10]

Finally, informed consent is required of all patients undergoing skin testing. Patients who decide to undergo in vivo testing must accept the discomforts of testing and risks of an adverse reaction and be willing to stop antihistamine medications or other medications that have relative contraindications during testing such as β-blocking medications. For patients who are either ineligible for in vivo testing or are unwilling to accept the risks and discomforts of in vivo testing, in vitro testing can be performed without the risks, discomfort, or other factors that preclude in vivo testing.

IN VITRO TESTING METHODS

In vitro testing consists of immunoassays that quantify the amount of serum-derived specific IgE binding to an allergen.[11] In vitro testing is the safest method for testing and can be performed in all patients who do not qualify for in vivo testing or who choose to undergo a safer means of allergen identification. In vitro testing is beneficial for patients who may be at a high risk for anaphylaxis, although this method of testing is less sensitive than skin testing.[4] Patients are also able to continue taking many of their medications such as antihistamines that are typically contraindicated in patients undergoing skin testing.[4]

The first available assay used radioactive anti-IgE to identify IgE in serum (radioallergosorbent test [RAST]).[12] The RAST assay was developed in 1972 with the commercially available Phadebas RAST and PRIST tests[10] that measured specific IgE compared with total serum IgE. The RAST assay used an isotopic to both identify and quantify antibodies present in sera. The components of the RAST assay, commonly referred to as *the sandwich assay*, consist of allergens attached to a base to form an immunosorbent particle. This immunosorbent particle binds with the designated IgE antibody creating an immune complex. The IgE antibody contains an Fc receptor that binds with the labeled IgE antigen. The combined antigen-antibody complex remaining after the rinsing process allows for quantification of specific IgE.[10] The modified RAST test was created in 1979 to increase the sensitivity of the RAST without compromising the specificity.

Newer technologies have replaced RAST owing to automatization and improved testing results. The newer technologies use enzymatic reactions (enzyme-linked immunosorbent assay) to produce a chemiluminescent, colorimetric, or fluorimetric reaction, the results of which are automated by a reader.[5,9,13] Currently available tests are approved by the US Food and Drug Administration and are standardized to a World Health Organization IgE standard.[14] The 3 autoanalyzer mechanisms most commonly used to quantify IgE are ImmunoCAP (Phadia AB, Uppsala, Sweden), Immulite (Siemens AG, Berlin, Germany), and HYTEC-288 (Hycor/Agilent, Garden Grove, CA); however, there are at least 15 different assays approved for use by the US Food and Drug Administration.[10,11] There are differences between each of the assays, and it is possible for 2 different assays to provide discordant results when analyzing the same antigen.[10]

In vitro testing has the advantage of providing quantitative results that can be used for treatment. Specific IgE levels correlate with the severity of symptoms and have been used to plan immunotherapy and predict response to desensitization.[15–20]

The results of in vitro testing depend somewhat on the quality of the testing laboratory. The IgE antibodies within the testing solution should only bind to its specific immunoglobulin class[10] and should not have any cross-reactivity with IgG antibodies. A high level of total IgE should not impact the measurement of specific IgE antibodies as has been reported.[10] Unfortunately, there is some variability in testing results because of the assay chosen and the laboratory evaluating the sample. Specific IgE testing results can vary between testing laboratory and technologies. A study comparing blinded samples of the same sera with those of multiple laboratories found less than half showed precision and accuracy in their results.[21] There has also been reported a poor agreement between results from different commercially available assays.[22,23] More recent technologies, such as the Immunocap ISAC, were studied at 23 sites and found consistency between sites with variability estimated at 25.5%.[24]

TOTAL IgE

Measurement of total serum IgE can provide clinically useful information.[2,25] When total IgE is low or not measureable, there is a low probability that in vitro–specific IgE results will be positive.[25] If allergy disease is suspected, alternative, more sensitive skin testing methods can be performed. Conversely, a high total IgE level in a patient with clinical symptoms is more likely to show sensitizations on in vitro testing.[2,25] Total serum IgE level can also help determine a patient's overall sensitivity and risks for anaphylaxis with exposure during testing and desensitization.

The total IgE level measurement in the serum is not always reliable, as there are various factors that can impact these levels, and it is still possible to have low total IgE levels with a positive allergy testing result.[2] There are other diseases with high total IgE that may not represent allergic sensitization to inhalant allergens. Evaluation of the IgE levels in patients with allergic diseases can be challenging, as they may already have high total IgE levels, and the response that they have to allergens could be low grade.[4] When the total serum IgE level is greatly increased, but the specific IgE testing negative, a false-negative result or alternative allergen that was not in the testing panel needs to be considered.

COMPARISON OF IN VIVO AND IN VITRO TESTING

Direct comparison of in vivo and in vitro allergy testing methods is challenging because of the different sensitizations within individuals, the range of severity of sensitivities, and the multiple methods for testing that continue to evolve with in vitro technologies.

Pumhirun and colleagues[19] studied specific IgE, skin prick, and intradermal testing for 2 dust mites. Sensitivities for skin prick tests were 90% and 86%, and specificities were 99% and 93%, respectively.[19] Sensitivities and specificities to *Dermatophagoides pteronyssinus* and *Dermatophagoides farinae* using specific IgE assay were both 96% and 89%, respectively.[19] This report shows the accuracy of in vitro testing for dust mites. In contrast, Chinoy and colleagues[26] and compared in vitro testing with skin testing using 4 indoor allergens and found skin testing to be more sensitive than RAST testing with poor correlation between the 2 methods.

Wood and colleagues[27] compared 3 testing methods for cat with 69% sensitivity and 100% specificity for in vitro testing with minimal additional benefits to intradermal testing over skin prick testing.[28] Tschopp and colleagues[29] compared in vitro testing with skin prick testing and found in vitro testing to be more sensitive but skin prick testing was more efficient. Bernstein and colleagues[6] reported a review of sensitivities for in vitro testing ranging from 50% to 90% with an average of 70% to 75%.

Some of the older data with early RAST is not as applicable today because of the improvement in accuracy with in vitro technologies.[30–32] More recently, Ferastraoaru and colleagues[33] compared intradermal and in vitro testing after negative skin prick testing and found that intradermal testing found 24% additional sensitization, whereas in vitro testing found only 9% additional sensitizations. There were instances in which in vitro results were positive (3%) despite negative skin prick and intradermal tests.

Intradermal testing results were positive (15%) when both other methods of testing had negative results. Nam and Lee[34] reported on comparison of skin prick test and serum-specific IgE to 17 common inhalant allergens. Agreement between the skin prick testing (SPT) and sIgE level was 75%. Overall agreement was moderate ($\kappa = 0.59$), with strong agreement for house dust mites and birch and weak agreement for *Tyrophagus putrescentiae* and dog.[34]

Overall, there is a wide range of sensitivity for in vitro testing with reported sensitivities between 67%and 96% and specificities between 80% and 100%.[19,28–31,33,34] Skin prick is more sensitive than in vitro testing by about 25%, which is beneficial as a screening method when clinical factors allow.[1,6,11,30] On the other hand, in vitro testing results in fewer false-positive results,[10] resulting in higher specificity.

For initiation of immunotherapy, the clinical information regarding the degree of individual sensitivity can help expedite treatment while reducing the risk of adverse reaction. In vitro testing allows for quantitative assessment of sensitization but does not measure the personal sensitivity upon exposure that is learned with skin testing. Initiation of immunotherapy based on in vitro testing should account for the possibility that a patient is more sensitive to exposure and thus the starting dose may be lower.

Although there are both benefits and limitations to in vivo and in vitro testing, there are clinical scenarios in which one method is preferred. The clinical factors also need to include a discussion with the patient regarding risks and benefits of each method so that patients can make an informed decision.

SUMMARY

Diagnoses and treatments of allergic rhinitis require a dynamic clinical assessment with multiple options for allergy testing. The patient history and physical examination should guide the need for diagnostic testing, type of diagnostic testing, and the interpretation of results. There are benefits to both in vivo and in vitro testing that must match the clinical scenario for each patient.

REFERENCES

1. Seidman MD, Gurgel RK, Lin SY, et al. Clinical practice guideline: allergic rhinitis. Otolaryngol Head Neck Surg 2015;152:S1–43.
2. Krouse J, Stachler R, Shah A. Current in vivo and in vitro screens for inhalant allergy. Otolaryngol Clin North Am 2003;36:855–68.
3. Rueff F, Bergmann K, Brockow K, et al. Skin tests for diagnostics of allergic immediate-type reactions. Guideline of the German Society for Allergology and Clinical Immunology. Pneumologie 2011;65(2):484–95.
4. Douglass J, OHehir R. Diagnosis, treatment and prevention of allergic disease: the basics. Med J Aust 2006;185(4):228–33.
5. Casset A, Khayah N, de Blay F. How in vitro assays contribute to allergy diagnosis. Curr Allergy Asthma Rep 2016;16:82.
6. Berstein IL, Li JT, Bernstein DI, et al. Allergy diagnostic testing: an updated practice parameter. Ann Allergy Asthma Immunol 2008;100(3 Suppl 3):S1–148.
7. Peltier J, Ryan M. Comparison of intradermal dilutional testing, skin prick testing, and modified quantitative testing for common allergens. Otolaryngol Head Neck Surg 2007;137(2):246–9.
8. Seshul M, Pillsbury H 3rd, Eby T. Use of intradermal dilutional testing and skin prick testing: clinical relevance and cost efficiency. Laryngoscope 2006;116(9): 1530–8.

9. Hamilton RG. Clinical laboratory assessment of immediate-type hypersensitivity. J Allergy Clin Immunol 2010;125(2 Suppl 2):S284–96.
10. Emanuel I. In vitro testing for allergy diagnosis. Otolaryngol Clin North Am 2003; 36:879–93.
11. Siles R, Hsieh F. Allergy blood testing: a practical guide for clinicians. Cleve Clin J Med 2011;78(9):585–92.
12. Krouse JH, Mabry RL. Skin testing for inhalant allergy 2003: current strategies. Otolaryngol Head Neck Surg 2003;129(4 Suppl):S33–49.
13. Cox L. Overview of serological-specific IgE antibody testing in children. Curr Allergy Asthma Rep 2011;11:447–53.
14. Osguthorpe JD. In vitro allergy testing. Int Forum Allergy Rhinol 2014;4:S46–50.
15. Corsico AG, De Amici M, Ronzoni V, et al. Allergen-specific immunoglobulin E and allergic rhinitis severity. Allergy Rhinol (Providence) 2017;1:1–4.
16. Chen ST, Sun HL, Lu KH, et al. Correlation of immunoglobulin E, eosinophil cationic protein, and eosinophil count with the severity of childhood perennial allergic rhinitis. J Microbiol Immunol Infect 2006;39:212–8.
17. Ciprandi G, De Amici M, Giunta V, et al. Comparison of serum specific IgE and skin prick test in polysensitized patients. Int J Immunopathol Pharmacol 2010; 23:1292–5.
18. Ciprandi G, Comite P, Ferrero F, et al. Serum allergen-specific IgE, allergic rhinitis severity, and age. Rhinology 2016;54:231–8.
19. Pumhirun P, Jane-Trakoonroj S, Wasuwat P. Comparison of in vitro assay for specific IgE and skin prick test with intradermal test in patients with allergic rhinitis. Asian Pac J Allergy Immunol 2000;18:157–60.
20. Howarth P, Malling HJ, Molimard M, et al. Analysis of allergen immunotherapy studies shows increased clinical efficacy in highly symptomatic patients. Allergy 2012;67:321–7.
21. Williams PB, Barnes JH, Szeinbach SL, et al. Analytic precision and accuracy of commercial immunoassays for specific IgE: establishing a standard. J Allergy Clin Immunol 2000;105:1221–30.
22. Wood R, Segall N, Ahlstedt S, et al. Accuracy of IgE antibody laboratory results. Ann Allergy 2007;99:34–41.
23. Wang J, Godbold JH, Sampson HA. Correlation of serum allergy (IgE) tests performed by different assay systems. J Allergy Clin Immunol 2008;121:1219–24.
24. van Hage M, Schmid-Grendelmeier P, Skevaki C, et al. Performance evaluation of ImmunoCAP ISAC 112: a multi-site study. Clin Chem Lab Med 2007;55:571–7.
25. Chung D, Park KT, Yarlagadda B, et al. The significance of serum total immunoglobulin E for in vitro diagnosis of allergic rhinitis. Int Forum Allergy Rhinol 2014; 4(1):56–60.
26. Chinoy B, Yee E, Bahna SL. Skin testing versus radioallergosorbent testing for indoor allergens. Clin Mol Allergy 2005;3:4.
27. Wood PA, Phipatanakul W, Hamilton RG, et al. A comparison of skin prick tests, intradermal skin tests, and RASTs in the diagnosis of cat allergy. J Allergy Clin Immunol 1999;103:773–9.
28. Ciprandi G, Comite P, Ferrero F, et al. Birch allergy and oral allergy syndrome: the practical relevance of serum IgE to Bet v 1. Allergy Asthma Proc 2016;37:43–9.
29. Tschopp J, Sistek D, Schindler C, et al. Current allergic asthma and rhinitis: diagnostic efficiency of three commonly used atopic markers (IgE, skin prick tests, and Phadiatop). Results from 8329 randomized adults from the SAPALDIA Study. Swiss study on Air Pollution and Lung Diseases in Adults. Allergy 1998;53: 608–13.

30. Ownby DR, Bailey J. Comparison of MAST with radioallergosorbent and skin test for diagnosis of allergy in children. Am J Dis Child 1986;140:45–8.
31. Ferguson AC, Murray AB. Predictive value of skin prick tests and radioallergosorbent tests for clinical allergy to dogs and cats. CMAJ 1986;134:1365–8.
32. Reddy PM, Nagaya H, Pascual HC, et al. Reappraisal of intracutaneous tests in the diagnosis of reaginic allergy. J Allergy Clin Immunol 1978;61:36–41.
33. Ferastraoaru D, Shtessel M, Lobell E, et al. Diagnosing environmental allergies: comparison of skin-prick, intradermal, and serum specific immunoglobulin E testing. Allergy Rhinol (Providence) 2017;8(2):53–62.
34. Nam YH, Lee SK. Comparison between skin prick test and serum immunoglobulin E by CAP system to inhalant allergens. Ann Allergy Asthma Immunol 2017; 118(5):608–13.

Efficacy and Safety of Subcutaneous and Sublingual Immunotherapy for Allergic Rhinoconjunctivitis and Asthma

Christopher R. Roxbury, MD, Sandra Y. Lin, MD*

KEYWORDS

- Subcutaneous immunotherapy • Sublingual immunotherapy • Allergic rhinitis
- Allergen-specific immunotherapy

KEY POINTS

- Allergen-specific immunotherapy is the only therapeutic option that may alter the course of allergic rhinitis and provide symptomatic relief after discontinuation of therapy.
- Immunotherapy may be offered in either subcutaneous or sublingual formulations.
- Current evidence supports subcutaneous immunotherapy as the gold standard for treatment of allergic rhinoconjunctivitis and asthma.
- Sublingual immunotherapy is found to be safe and is an effective alternative therapy for patients unable to tolerate injections, who cannot make frequent trips to the physician's office, or who desire an alternative to injection immunotherapy.

INTRODUCTION

Allergic rhinitis (AR) is caused by a type 1, IgE-mediated immediate hypersensitivity reaction in the nasal mucosa in response to inhaled environmental allergens, with prevalence estimates between 10% and 20% in US adults and slightly higher prevalence in children.[1–3] As a result, patients may experience a combination of symptoms including nasal itching, sneezing, and nasal congestion. Additionally, these patients often experience comorbid allergic conjunctivitis and asthma. Although these sequelae are not dangerous, they can have a profound impact on quality of life,

Disclosure Statement: The authors have no financial conflicts of interest to disclose.
Department of Otolaryngology–Head and Neck Surgery, Johns Hopkins University School of Medicine, 601 North Caroline Street, 6th Floor, Baltimore, MD 21287, USA
* Corresponding author. Department of Otolaryngology–Head and Neck Surgery, Johns Hopkins Outpatient Center, 601 North Caroline Street, 6th Floor, Baltimore, MD 21287.
E-mail address: slin30@jhmi.edu

leading to decreased productivity at school and work.[4,5] Moreover, AR has been shown to have a significant financial impact in the United States, with indirect costs being estimated as high as $9.7 billion.[6] Asthma is often seen in conjunction with AR, as 62% of patients with asthma have a history of atopy.[7]

Management of AR consists of avoidance of environmental allergens, pharmacotherapy, and allergen-specific immunotherapy (AIT). Specifics of allergen avoidance and pharmacotherapy are beyond the scope of this article. Although most patients do well with avoidance measures and pharmacotherapy alone, AIT is the only definitive therapy available that may alter the natural history of disease. This therapy involves repetitive dosing of allergens in a controlled fashion, with the ultimate goal of increasing tolerance to the allergen, decreasing AR symptoms, and reducing the need for pharmacotherapy.

There are currently 2 forms of AIT available in the United States: subcutaneous immunotherapy (SCIT) and sublingual immunotherapy (SLIT),[8] which may be offered to patients with AR symptoms and positive allergy skin testing. Compared with SCIT, which involves repeat office visits and injections, SLIT involves introduction of allergen tablets or aqueous drops under the tongue. As such, SLIT may provide a simpler and easier-to-deliver form of AIT. Although the US Food and Drug Administration has only recently approved tablet formulations of SLIT, as of 2009, up to 80% of all AIT in Europe consisted of SLIT.[9] In addition, the off-label use of aqueous SCIT allergens for SLIT in the United States has also been increasing in popularity.[10] The objective of this review is to compare subcutaneous and sublingual immunotherapy in terms of clinical efficacy and safety profile (**Table 1**).

SUBCUTANEOUS IMMUNOTHERAPY
Dosing and Patient Considerations

SCIT was first described in 1911[11] and remains the mainstay of AIT performed in the United States. Subcutaneous immunotherapy is indicated in individuals with positive allergy skin testing and allergic rhinitis with poorly controlled symptoms using maximal pharmacotherapy and in patients with coexisting allergy and asthma. Relative indications include inability to tolerate pharmacotherapy or desire to avoid the need for pharmacotherapy.[12,13]

SCIT may be performed in the setting of previous quantitative skin testing, whereby a safe starting dose of antigen is determined. The initial dose is gradually increased during the escalation phase of SCIT, in which weekly injections are performed with the goal of reaching a maintenance dose that appropriately alleviates AR symptoms without adverse effects. Maintenance doses depend on patient factors such as ability to tolerate injections and compliance. There are known ranges for effective doses of dust mite, cat, dog, pooid grasses, and ragweed allergens.[13] When an effective dose is reached, a maintenance phase of 3 to 5 years of regularly scheduled injections is typically initiated.[14]

Effectiveness

The World Allergy Organization (WAO) recommends that the minimum clinically relevant efficacy of immunotherapy be "at least 20% higher than placebo."[15] Several randomized, controlled trials and systematic reviews assessed the efficacy of SCIT. High-grade evidence suggests that SCIT is effective in improving symptoms of asthma and rhinoconjunctivitis, decreasing asthma medication usage, and improving disease-specific quality of life in patients with rhinitis/rhinoconjunctivitis.[16–23] There is moderate evidence to suggest SCIT decreases medication use in rhinoconjunctivitis. The

Table 1
Comparison of subcutaneous and sublingual immunotherapy for allergic rhinoconjunctivitis and asthma

	SCIT	SLIT
Dosing	Physician office visits for repeat injections required, 3- to 5-y treatment period effective.	Patient may administer sublingual drops at home, >5-y treatment period likely most effective.
Safety		
Local reactions	Local reactions (skin pruritus) reported in up to 58% of patients or 10% of injections.	Local reactions (pruritus, floor of mouth edema) reported in up to 97% of patients.
Systemic reactions	Systemic reactions (respiratory symptoms) may occur in up to 71% of patients or 27% of injections. Fatalities may occur in up to 1 in 25 million injection visits.	One case of anaphylaxis reported in 1 billion administrations. No fatalities reported.
Effectiveness		
Allergic rhinitis and rhinoconjunctivitis	Evidence from systematic reviews to support improved symptoms, medication scores, and quality of life.	Evidence from systematic reviews to support improved symptoms, medication scores, and quality of life.
Asthma	Evidence from randomized controlled trials to support dust mite SCIT in the treatment of allergic asthma in children.	Little evidence to support use of SLIT for treatment of adult asthma. Evidence from systematic reviews and meta-analyses to support improved symptom and medication scores, and decreased asthma severity with dust mite SLIT in children.

effectiveness of SCIT on allergic rhinitis/rhinoconjunctivitis and asthma is discussed further later in this report.

Allergic rhinitis/rhinoconjunctivitis

There is strong evidence suggesting that SCIT improves symptoms, medication use, and quality of life in patients with allergic rhinoconjunctivitis. A systematic review assessing effectiveness of SCIT for allergic conjunctivitis found moderate-to-strong evidence to support symptomatic improvement in allergic rhinitis and asthma. Eleven studies assessed conjunctivitis symptoms in 889 patients, 10 of which found greater improvement in symptoms with SCIT compared with controls.[21] A meta-analysis both directly and indirectly comparing SCIT with SLIT using data from 17 SCIT randomized controlled trials and 11 SLIT randomized controlled trials showed no statistically significant difference in quality of life between the modalities.[24]

More recently, a systematic review from Europe analyzed 61 SCIT randomized controlled studies including 6379 patients. Most of the studies included in this review reported on short-term effectiveness in primarily adult patients, with multiple allergens studied. The results of this systematic review suggest strong evidence that SCIT improves short-term symptom control, decreases need for medications, and increases disease-specific quality of life in patients with allergic rhinoconjunctivitis, with modest evidence for long-term improvement in symptom scores after discontinuation of therapy.[22]

Asthma

The preponderance of evidence regarding the use of SCIT for asthma comes from randomized controlled trials of dust mite SCIT. Of 10 previous studies assessing asthma symptoms, 9 showed significant improvement of allergy symptoms with SCIT.[21] Of 8 studies assessing asthma medication use, 5 showed a significant decrease in need for asthma medication with SCIT.[21] When assessing bronchial reactivity after specific allergen challenge, 8 of 11 (72.7%) studies found statistically significant improvement after SCIT, but results were inconsistent in 11 studies assessing pulmonary function tests.[21] For these reasons, several guidelines recommend dust mite SCIT as an effective option for allergic asthma,[25–27] although there is no consensus on the use SCIT in asthma therapy in adults.[28] There is more support for dust mite SCIT in children, as there is evidence suggesting that allergy plays a stronger role in childhood asthma.[26]

Safety

Adverse reactions to SCIT range from local site reactions such as skin pruritus to systemic reactions such as anaphylaxis and have been previously classified by the WAO.[29] Rates of local reactions are reported to be between 5% and 58% of patients and 3% and 10% of injections. The most common systemic reactions reported are respiratory in nature and occur in up to 71% of patients or 27% of injections.[23] Patients with a history of systemic reactions may be 4 times as likely to experience a systemic reaction as those with no history of systemic reaction.[30] A survey of fatal SCIT reactions performed between 1990 and 2001 reported 41 fatalities associated with SCIT, or a rate of 1 death per every 25 million injection visits.[31] Upon further review of 17 of these cases, 15 (88.2%) occurred in patients with uncontrolled asthma. A further survey conducted between 2008 and 2013 found 2 direct reports of fatalities in patients treated by allergists and 2 indirect reports of fatalities in patients under the care of nonallergists, representing a significant decrease in injection-related deaths.[32] Thus, although SCIT is widely considered safe, there is potential for serious systemic reactions, particularly in patients at risk for systemic allergic response such as those with uncontrolled asthma.[33] Moreover, careful consideration should be given to the risk/benefit ratio of immunotherapy in those patients who are concomitantly taking a β-blocker, as more serious or treatment-resistant anaphylaxis may occur in these patients.[34] Because of concerns regarding SCIT safety, it is recommended that injections are performed in a physician's office and that the patient be monitored for 30 minutes for any adverse reactions.[34]

SUBLINGUAL IMMUNOTHERAPY
Dosing and Patient Considerations

Administration schedules for SLIT reported in the literature are more variable than with SCIT. Most recently, daily dosing has been used.[23] In contrast to SCIT, SLIT dosing is performed at home by the patient. A study of differing induction schedule lengths showed no difference in adverse events between 8-, 15- and 20-day inductions.[35] Escalation is typically rapid compared with SCIT, with no escalation being performed in European formulations that start with the maintenance dose. In the United States, sublingual grass tablets require no dose escalation in patients age 18 to 65 and a 3-day escalation for patients age 10 to 17.[36]

The duration of therapy in SLIT remains controversial. A previous trial of 3-, 4-, or 5-year duration of therapy with single-allergen SLIT reported improvements in AR symptoms for 7 years in those receiving treatment for 3 years and improvements for 8 years in those receiving a 4- or 5-year course.[37] Indeed, a recent double-blind, randomized, placebo-controlled trial failed to show any significant improvement in nasal response to allergen challenge over placebo in patients receiving 2 years of sublingual grass pollen immunotherapy,[38] suggesting that longer courses of therapy are likely needed. However, SLIT may still be an attractive option to patients who cannot tolerate frequent injections or who would prefer to avoid the inconvenience of frequent physician visits.

Effectiveness

Allergic rhinitis/rhinoconjunctivitis

SLIT is found to be effective in the management of allergic rhinitis by several systematic reviews,[19,20,39] with moderate evidence that SLIT improves symptoms of allergic rhinitis/rhinoconjunctivitis and decreases medication use.[39] Other systematic reviews found that SLIT with grass and dust mite allergens also improves symptoms in these patients.[40,41] Some suggest that SLIT may be an attractive alternative to SCIT in the pediatric population because of increased patient compliance in the setting of avoiding injections. In a meta-analysis of 9 pediatric studies included in a Cochrane review, SLIT was proven effective for symptomatic improvement.[42] The previously mentioned systematic review by Dhami and colleagues[22] compared SLIT in adults and children and found that short-term symptom and medication scores were improved in both groups. Although a previous analysis of 4 systematic reviews suggested that SCIT is more effective than SLIT at decreasing allergic rhinoconjunctivitis symptoms and reducing the need for medication,[43] SLIT was also compared with SCIT in several outcomes by Dhami, and colleagues[22] including short-term improvement in symptom scores, medication scores, and combined symptom and medication scores. This large meta-analysis of 160 studies showed no significant differences between the 2 modalities.

Asthma

Strong evidence supports the use of SLIT for symptomatic improvement in allergic asthma,[39] with several reports specifically studying the effectiveness of SLIT on asthma in children. Two meta-analyses found that SLIT may improve symptoms and medication use in children with asthma,[44,45] whereas other studies found that dust mite SLIT may decrease severity of asthma,[46] and grass pollen SLIT may make children 3.8 times less likely to have asthma.[47] There are little data regarding the use of SLIT for asthma in adults, although there are low-grade data to suggest that SCIT is more effective than SLIT for improvement of asthma symptoms.[48]

Safety

Overall, SLIT is found to have a better safety profile than SCIT. However, adverse reactions are possible just as they are with SCIT. The most common adverse reactions are mucosal pruritus and irritation at the site of administration in the oral cavity. Gastrointestinal upset, nausea, vomiting, and diarrhea have also been reported and are considered local reactions by the WAO.[49] A review of SLIT safety performed in 2006 showed a rate of 14 systemic adverse reactions in 1 million administrations,[50] and a systematic review of randomized controlled trials performed in 2013 showed no reported cases of anaphylaxis, although rates of local reactions with SLIT were as high as 97%.[23] Although the studies included in this review did not report anaphylaxis, another review reported 1 case of anaphylaxis in 1 billion SLIT doses,[51] and another recent study reported a case of a WAO grade 2 systemic reaction requiring intramuscular epinephrine in a patient receiving timothy grass SLIT.[52] In the GRASS study, among 36 patients receiving SLIT over 2 years, there were no systemic reactions requiring the use of epinephrine.[38] Thus, although SLIT seems to be safe, it is recommended that the first dose of SLIT be administered in the physician's office, and an epinephrine autoinjector should be prescribed for use while home administration of SLIT is performed. Moreover, just as with SCIT, SLIT should not be administered in patients with severe or uncontrolled asthma or history of previous systemic allergic reactions.

SUMMARY

Allergen immunotherapy is the only treatment that may affect the natural course of disease in AR and asthma and may lead to symptomatic benefits even after discontinuation of therapy. Although SCIT remains the gold standard for AIT, it is not without drawbacks including the need for repeat physician office visits, injections, and risk for systemic allergic reactions. There is a growing body of literature to support SLIT as a safe and effective alternative therapy for appropriately selected patients with AR or asthma. Further studies are needed to assess the efficacy of multiple-allergen SLIT and to determine optimal dosing induction and maintenance schedules.

REFERENCES

1. Salo PM, Calatroni A, Gergen PJ, et al. Allergy-related outcomes in relation to serum IgE: results from the National Health and Nutrition Examination Survey 2005–2006. J Allergy Clin Immunol 2011;127:1226–35.e7.
2. Mims JW. Epidemiology of allergic rhinitis. Int Forum Allergy Rhinol 2014;4: S18–20.
3. Wright AL, Holberg CJ, Martinez FD, et al. Epidemiology of physiciandiagnosed allergic rhinitis in childhood. Pediatrics 1994;94(6 Pt 1):895–901.
4. Meltzer EO, Blaiss MS, Derebery MJ, et al. Burden of allergic rhinitis: results from the pediatric allergies in America survey. J Allergy Clin Immunol 2009;124(3 Suppl):S43–70.
5. Meltzer EO, Nathan R, Derebery J, et al. Sleep, quality of life, and productivity impact of nasal symptoms in the United States: findings from the burden of rhinitis in America survey. Allergy Asthma Proc 2009;30:244–54.
6. Reed SD, Lee TA, McCrory DC. The economic burden of allergic rhinitis: a critical evaluation of the literature. Pharmacoeconomics 2004;22:345–61.
7. Gergen PJ, Arbes SJ Jr, Calatroni A, et al. Total IgE levels and asthma prevalence in the US population: results from the National Health and Nutrition Examination Survey 2005–2006. J Allergy Clin Immunol 2009;124:447–53.
8. Lin SY. Sublingual immunotherapy: current concepts for the U.S. practitioner. Int Forum Allergy Rhinol 2014;4:S55–9.
9. Cox L, Jacobsen L. Comparison of allergen immunotherapy practice patterns in the United States and Europe. Ann Allergy Asthma Immunol 2009;103(6):451–9.
10. Ryan MW, Marple BF, Leatherman B, et al. Current practice trends in allergy: results of a united states survey of otolaryngologists, allergist-immunologists, and primary care physicians. Int Forum Allergy Rhinol 2014;4(10):789–95.
11. Noon L. Prophylactic inoculation against hay fever. Lancet 1911;177:1572–3.
12. Joint Task Force on Practice Parameters, American Academy of Allergy, Asthma and Immunology, American College of Allergy, Asthma and Immunology, Joint Council of Allergy, Asthma and Immunology. Allergen immunotherapy: a practice parameter second update. J Allergy Clin Immunol 2007;120(3 Suppl):S25–85.

13. Seidman MD, Gurgel RK, Lin SY, et al. Clinical practice guideline: allergic rhinitis. Otolaryngol Head Neck Surg 2015;152(1 Suppl):S1–43.
14. Roche AM, Wise SK. Subcutaneous immunotherapy. Int Forum Allergy Rhinol 2014;4:S51–4.
15. Canonica GW, Baena-Cagnani CE, Bousquet J, et al. Recommendations for standardization of clinical trials with allergen specific immunotherapy for respiratory allergy. A statement of a World Allergy Organization (WAO) taskforce. Allergy 2007;62:317–24.
16. Matricardi PM, Kuna P, Panetta V, et al. Subcutaneous immunotherapy and pharmacotherapy in seasonal allergic rhinitis: a comparison based on metaanalyses. J Allergy Clin Immunol 2011;128:791–9.e6.
17. Calderon MA, Alves B, Jacobson M, et al. Allergen injection immunotherapy for seasonal allergic rhinitis. Cochrane Database Syst Rev 2007;(1):CD001936.
18. Abramson MJ, Puy RM, Weiner JM. Injection allergen immunotherapy for asthma. Cochrane Database Syst Rev 2010;(8):CD001186.
19. Wilson DR, Torres LI, Durham SR. Sublingual immunotherapy for allergic rhinitis. Cochrane Database Syst Rev 2003;(2):CD002893.
20. Radulovic S, Wilson D, Calderon M, et al. Systematic reviews of sublingual immunotherapy (SLIT). Allergy 2011;66:740–52.
21. Erekosima N, Suarez-Cuervo C, Ramanathan M, et al. Effectiveness of subcutaneous immunotherapy for allergic rhinoconjunctivitis and asthma: a systematic review. Laryngoscope 2014;124(3):616–27.
22. Dhami S, Nurmatov U, Arasi S, et al. Allergen immunotherapy for allergic rhinoconjunctivitis: a systematic review and meta-analysis. Allergy 2017. http://dx.doi.org/10.1111/all.13201.
23. Lin SY, Erekosima N, Suarez-Cuervo C, et al. Allergen-specific immunotherapy for the treatment of allergic rhinoconjunctivitis and/or asthma: comparative effectiveness review. Rockville (MD): Agency for Healthcare Research and Quality; 2013. Comparative effectiveness review No. 111. (Prepared by the Johns Hopkins University evidence-based practice center under contract No. 290-2007-10061-I.) AHRQ publication No. 13-EHC061-EF.
24. Dretzke J, Meadows A, Novielli N, et al. Subcutaneous and sublingual immunotherapy for seasonal allergic rhinitis: a systematic review and indirect comparison. J Allergy Clin Immunol 2013;131:1361–6.
25. National Asthma Education and Prevention Program. Expert panel report 3 (EPR-3): guidelines for the diagnosis and management of asthma-summary report 2007. J Allergy Clin Immunol 2007;120:S94–138.
26. Papadopoulos N, Arakawa H, Carlsen KH, et al. International consensus on (ICON) pediatric asthma. Allergy 2012;67:976–97.
27. Motala C, Green RJ, Manjra A, et al. Guideline for the management of chronic asthma in children-2009 update. S Afr Med J 2009;99:898–912.
28. Calderón MA, Bousquet J, Canonica GW, et al. Guideline recommendations on the use of allergen immunotherapy in house dust mite allergy: time for a change? J Allergy Clin Immunol 2017;140(1):41–52.
29. Cox L, Larenas-Linnemann D, Lockey RF, et al. Speaking the same language: the World Allergy Organization subcutaneous immunotherapy systemic reaction grading system. J Allergy Clin Immunol 2010;125:569–74.
30. Roy SR, Sigmon JR, Olivier J, et al. Increased frequency of large local reactions among systemic reactors during subcutaneous allergen immunotherapy. Ann Allergy Asthma Immunol 2007;99:82–6.

31. Bernstein DI, Wanner M, Borish L, et al. Twelve-year survey of fatal reactions to allergen injections and skin testing: 1990-2001. J Allergy Clin Immunol 2004; 113:1129–36.

32. Epstein TG, Liss GM, Murphy-Berendts K, et al. Risk factors for fatal and nonfatal reactions to subcutaneous immunotherapy: national surveillance study on allergen immunotherapy (2008–2013). Ann Allergy Asthma Immunol 2016;116: 354–9.

33. James C, Bernstein DI. Allergen immunotherapy: an updated review of safety. Curr Opin Allergy Clin Immuno 2017;17(1):55–9.

34. Cox L, Lockey R, Nelson H, et al. Allergen immunotherapy: a practice parameter third update. J Allergy Clin Immunol 2011;127(1):S1–55.

35. Sambugaro R, Puccinelli P, Burastero SE, et al. The efficacy of sublingual immunotherapy for respiratory allergy is not affected by different dosage regimens in the induction phase. Allergol Immunopathol (Madr) 2003;31:329–37.

36. Oralair package insert. Available at: http://www.fda.gov/downloads/ BiologicsBloodVaccines/Allergenics/UCM391580.pdf. Accessed May 22, 2016.

37. Marogna M, Spadolini I, Massolo A, et al. Longlasting effect of sublingual immunotherapy according to its duration: a 15 year prospective study. J Allergy Clin Immunol 2010;126:969–75.

38. Scadding GW, Calderon MA, Shamji MH, et al. Effect of 2 years of treatment with sublingual grass pollen immunotherapy on nasal response to allergen challenge at 3 years among patients with moderate to severe seasonal allergic rhinitis: the grass randomized clinical trial. JAMA 2017;317(6):615–25.

39. Lin SY, Erekosima N, Kim JM, et al. Sublingual immunotherapy for the treatment of allergic rhinoconjunctivitis and asthma: a systematic review. JAMA 2013;309: 1278–88.

40. Di Bona D, Plaia A, Scafidi V, et al. Efficacy of sublingual immunotherapy with grass allergens for seasonal allergic rhinitis: a systematic review and meta-analysis. J Allergy Clin Immunol 2010;126:558–66.

41. Compalati E, Passalacqua G, Bonini M, et al. The efficacy of sublingual immunotherapy for house dust mites respiratory allergy: results of a GA2LEN meta analysis. Allergy 2009;64:1570–9.

42. Calderon MA, Penagos M, Sheikh A, et al. Sublingual immunotherapy for allergic conjunctivitis: cochrane systematic review and meta-analysis. Clin Exp Allergy 2011;41:1263–72.

43. Chelladurai Y, Lin SY. Effectiveness of subcutaneous versus sublingual immunotherapy for allergic rhinitis: current update. Curr Opin Otolaryngol Head Neck Surg 2014;22:211–5.

44. Kim JM, Lin SY, Suarez-Cuervo C, et al. Allergen specific immunotherapy for pediatric asthma and rhinoconjunctivitis: a systematic review. Pediatrics 2013;131: 1155–67.

45. Penagos M, Passalacqua G, Compalati E, et al. Metaanalysis of the efficacy of sublingual immunotherapy in the treatment of allergic asthma in pediatric patients, 3 to 18 years of age. Chest 2008;133:599–609.

46. Marogna M, Tomassetti D, Bernasconi A, et al. Preventive effects of sublingual immunotherapy in childhood: an open randomized controlled study. Ann Allergy Asthma Immunol 2008;101:206–11.

47. Novembre E, Galli E, Landi F, et al. Coseasonal sublingual immunotherapy reduces the development of asthma in children with allergic rhinoconjunctivitis. J Allergy Clin Immunol 2004;114:851–7.

48. Chelladurai Y, Suarez-Cuervo C, Erekosima N, et al. Effectiveness of subcutaneous versus sublingual immunotherapy for the treatment of allergic rhinoconjunctivitis and asthma: a systematic review. J Allergy Clin Immunol Pract 2013;1(4): 361–9.
49. Canonica GW, Cox L, Pawankar R, et al. Sublingual immunotherapy: World Allergy Organization position paper 2013 update. World Allergy Organ J 2014;7:6.
50. Cox LS, Linnemann DL, Nolte H, et al. Sublingual immunotherapy: a comprehensive review. J Allergy Clin Immunol 2006;117:1021–35.
51. Calderon MA, Simons FER, Malling HJ, et al. Sublingual allergen immunotherapy: mode of action and its relationship with the safety profile. Allergy 2012;67: 302–11.
52. Wasan A, Nanda A. Systemic reaction to timothy grass pollen sublingual immunotherapy. Ann Allergy Asthma Immunol 2017;118:732–3.

Clinical Applications of Sublingual Immunotherapy

Thomas S. Edwards, MD, Sarah K. Wise, MD, MSCR*

KEYWORDS

- Sublingual immunotherapy • Allergic rhinitis • Allergic asthma • Asthma
- Atopic dermatitis • Food allergy • Allergy • Immunotherapy

KEY POINTS

- Sublingual immunotherapy (SLIT) reduces symptoms and medication use in allergic rhinitis. Literature suggests that SLIT efficacy may persist for up to 8 years following a 4-year course of treatment.
- SLIT reduces the risk of moderate/severe allergic asthma exacerbations and is indicated in patients who remain symptomatic. Uncontrolled asthma is a contraindication for SLIT.
- Although additional studies are needed, SLIT is effective for some food allergies.
- In appropriately selected patients, SLIT safety profile is excellent. Anaphylaxis does occur, but at an estimated rate of 1 case per 100 million doses, the risk is exceedingly small.

INTRODUCTION

Approximately 25% of the population of the United States has an allergic disease, encompassing rhinitis, conjunctivitis, asthma, atopic dermatitis, urticaria, and food allergy.[1] Allergic rhinitis (AR) is the most common chronic childhood disease and the fifth most common overall; it is responsible for $3.4 billion in direct medical costs annually.[2,3] Asthma is also very common, with 7.8% of the US population and 300 million people worldwide affected.[4]

Allergy prevalence is increasing. The rates of AR, peanut allergy, and asthma have nearly doubled between 1980 and 2000.[1] The World Health Organization expects 100 million new asthma diagnoses in the next 10 years.[4] The hygiene hypothesis, recently retitled the microflora, biodiversity, or microbiome hypothesis, refers to microbiome disruption in childhood by antibiotic use as well as lifestyle, diet, and birth practice

Disclosures: None (T.S. Edwards). Medtronic–Consultant, Elron–Consultant (S.K. Wise).
Department of Otolaryngology–Head and Neck Surgery, Emory Sinus, Nasal and Allergy Center, Emory University, 550 Peachtree Street Northeast, MOT 11th Floor, Atlanta, GA 30308, USA
* Corresponding author.
E-mail address: skmille@emory.edu

Otolaryngol Clin N Am 50 (2017) 1121–1134
http://dx.doi.org/10.1016/j.otc.2017.08.010
0030-6665/17/© 2017 Elsevier Inc. All rights reserved.

changes, leading to an increased risk of allergic disease.[5-7] This hypothesis, coupled with worldwide development, are commonly implicated for rising allergy prevalence.[8]

More than one-third of patients with allergic syndromes remain undiagnosed or do not receive appropriate therapy.[1] Both physician-related and patient-related causes are implicated. Physicians often overlook allergy screening or overestimate the degree of control achieved with current therapy. Therefore, therapies are not escalated when treatment fails.[1] Often, patients do not seek medical care for AR. More than 50% of patients with uncontrolled AR symptoms had not seen a physician in the past year for treatment. Those who do seek care wait until symptoms are "intolerable."[9] Further, almost half of patients receiving specialist care report nonadherence.[1] Some patients avoid treatment due to medication cost or side effects, as well as unfounded concerns about the habit-forming nature of medications. The least common reason is lack of efficacy.[9]

In general, patients desire therapies that treat the root cause of their disease and provide lasting relief. Immunotherapy is the only disease-modifying and durable therapy for allergic disease. However, only 5% of eligible patients are offered allergy immunotherapy (AIT).[1]

AIT induces allergen tolerance by initially producing a population of $CD4^+CD25^+$ T lymphocytes (regulatory T cells) that secrete inhibitory cytokines (interleukin-10 and/or transforming growth factor-β). These cytokines decrease antigen-specific production of immunoglobulin (Ig)E by B cells; reduce proinflammatory cytokine release from mast cells, eosinophils, and T cells; and lead to tolerance of T cells by inhibiting the CD28 costimulatory pathway. Long-term AIT leads to a shift from a T_H2 to a T_H1 cytokine response.[10]

AIT was first described in 1900 for hay fever and used an oral ragweed extract.[11] Subcutaneous immunotherapy (SCIT) has traditionally been the favored route of AIT administration in the United States. However, following 26 SCIT-related anaphylaxis deaths in the United Kingdom, there was increased interest in alternative IT routes with improved safety profiles.[12] Aqueous allergen extracts are not currently approved by the US Food and Drug Administration (FDA) for sublingual immunotherapy (SLIT), but they are often used off-label by US practitioners. This review summarizes SLIT efficacy and safety for the treatment of several allergic diseases and provides tips for the practical implementation of SLIT.

SUBLINGUAL IMMUNOTHERAPY FOR ALLERGIC RHINITIS

AR is a IgE-mediated type I hypersensitivity reaction causing inflammation of the nasal mucosa with exposure to an inciting trigger. Characteristic symptoms include nasal congestion, rhinorrhea, and sneezing.[2] An estimated 500 million people worldwide have AR.[8,13] AR treatments include antihistamines, corticosteroids, leukotriene receptor antagonists, and AIT (SCIT and SLIT), among others. Only AIT alters the natural course of the disease.[2]

Indications and Contraindications

The American Academy of Otolaryngology–Head and Neck Surgery recommends "…immunotherapy (sublingual or subcutaneous) for patients with AR who have inadequate relief of symptoms with pharmacologic therapy…."[2] Many patients undergo empiric pharmacotherapy with intranasal corticosteroids, second-generation oral H_1-antihistamines, and/or intranasal H_1-antihistamines initially.[2]

Skin or in vitro allergy testing is often next undertaken in patients with AR. If results of allergy testing are positive, indicating type I IgE-mediated reactivity, an association between positive test allergens and symptom pattern should be confirmed and patients may be screened for suitability for AIT. Absolute contraindications to SLIT include history of severe local or systemic reaction to SLIT; severe, uncontrolled, or unstable asthma; current beta-blocker use (although some consider this a relative contraindication); hypersensitivity to an inactive ingredient in the SLIT preparation; and a history of eosinophilic esophagitis. Other considerations include patient compliance, other immunologic diseases, comorbidities, and cost (**Table 1**).[2,14–18] AIT can be continued in patients who become pregnant. Recent literature also suggests AIT may be safely initiated in pregnant patients.[19] Pediatric patients are candidates for AIT. SLIT studies included children as young as 4 years.[20]

Efficacy

Multiple large-scale systematic reviews and meta-analyses, including a Cochrane review of 60 double-blinded randomized controlled trials (DBRCTs), demonstrate SLIT efficacy for AR in adults and children (**Table 2**).[16,17,21,22] The Cochrane review found a significant reduction in symptoms (standardized mean difference [SMD] -0.49; 95% confidence interval (CI) -0.64 to -0.34, $P<.00001$) and medication requirements (SMD -0.32; 95% CI -0.43 to -0.21, $P<.00001$) in participants receiving SLIT versus placebo.[16] A more recent systematic review of 63 DBRCTs, considering an additional 11 studies not included in the Cochrane review, noted a moderate strength of evidence supporting SLIT for AR (rhinitis/rhinoconjunctivitis), with 4 studies demonstrating statistically significant improvements in disease-specific quality of life using validated instruments.[17]

The progression from atopic dermatitis (AD) to AR to allergic asthma (AA) is referred to as the "allergic march."[2] Some studies assert that AIT prevents the progression of AR to asthma. A 2013 systematic review of AIT for asthma and AR in pediatric patients included 3 studies that evaluated the prevention of asthma with SLIT.[20] Two studies showed decreased new asthma diagnoses in patients with AR treated with SLIT versus placebo.[23,24] One study showed children receiving conventional AR treatment were 3.8 times (95% CI 1.5–10.0) more likely to develop asthma versus those receiving SLIT for 3 years.[24] Another study evaluating SLIT treatment for 2 years, however, showed no difference in the number of patients with asthma at 8 years of follow-up.[25]

Four SLIT tablet formulations are currently approved by the US FDA for AR treatment. Timothy Grass Pollen Allergen Extract (Grastek; Merck), House Dust Mite (*Dermatophagoides farinae* and *Dermatophagoides pteronyssinus*) Allergen Extract Tablet for Sublingual Use (Odactra; Merck, Kenilworth, NJ, USA), a 5-grass tablet

Table 1

Indications, contraindications, and additional considerations to initiation of sublingual immunotherapy (SLIT)

Indications	Contraindications	Additional Considerations
• Failure of avoidance measures and pharmacotherapy • Evidence of immunoglobulin E–mediated disease via skin or in vitro testing • Association between reactive antigens and symptoms	• History of severe local or systemic reaction to SLIT • Severe, uncontrolled, or unstable asthma • History of eosinophilic esophagitis • Current use of β-blockers • Hypersensitivity to an inactive ingredient in the SLIT preparation	• Other immunologic disease • Social factors (eg, cost, concerns about patient adherence)

Table 2
Meta-analyses and systematic reviews of the efficacy of SLIT for AR

Citation	Included Studies	n	Results	Conclusion
Radulovic et al,[16] 2010	49	4589	Symptoms: SMD −0.49 95% CI −0.64 to −0.34 P<.00001 Medication Use: SMD −0.32 95% CI −0.43 to −0.21 P<.00001	"Sublingual immunotherapy is now established as a viable alternative to allergen injection immunotherapy, with a significantly lower risk profile and, on the basis of meta-analyses, little difference in overall efficacy."
Lin et al,[17] 2013	36	2985	• 94% of studies demonstrated greater improvement in the SLIT groups vs placebo. • Medium risk of bias. • Magnitude of association was moderate or strong in 14 studies (39%).	"…moderate strength in the evidence to support the use of sublingual immunotherapy for allergic rhinitis and asthma."
Devillier et al,[21] 2014	38	21,223	• Five-grass pollen SLIT tablets: Weighted mean RCI on symptom scores, (range) −29.6% (−23% to −37%) • Timothy pollen SLIT tablets: RCI −19.2% (−6% to −29%) • Nasal corticosteroids: RCI −23.5% (−7% to −54%) • Azelastine-fluticasone combination (MP29–02): RCI −17.1% (−15% to −20%) • H1-antihistamines: RCI -15.0% (−3% to −26%) • Montelukast RCI −6.5% (−3% to −10%)	"…grass pollen SLIT tablets [were] associated with a greater [RCI] than that provided by second-generation H1-antihistamines and a leukotriene receptor antagonist…"
Di Bona et al,[22] 2015	13	4659	Symptoms: SMD −0.28 95% CI, −0.37 to −0.19 P<.001 Medication Use: SMD −0.24 95% CI, −0.31 to −0.17 P<.001	"…small benefit of the grass pollen sublingual tablets in reducing symptoms and in decreasing the use of symptomatic medication…in patients with [seasonal allergic rhinoconjunctivitis]."

Abbreviations: CI, confidence interval; RCI, relative clinical impact; SLIT, sublingual immunotherapy; SMD, standardized mean difference.

(Sweet Vernal, Orchard, Perennial Rye, Timothy, and Kentucky Blue Grass Mixed Pollens Allergen Extract [Oralair; Stallergenes-Greer, Cambridge, MA, USA]), and Short Ragweed Pollen Allergen Extract (Ragwitek; Merck). Prescribing information and indications for these medications are slightly varied (**Table 3**).[26–29]

Durability

The reduction in AR symptoms begins from several weeks to 1 year after SLIT initiation.[2] Treatment effect may persist up to 8 years following SLIT completion, based on one study.[30] Although symptoms may return, a 15-year longitudinal study compared SLIT treatment length (3, 4, or 5 years) and showed a 4-year treatment course to be optimal. This study also showed a second SLIT course had prompt clinical impact after attenuation of the first course's benefit.[30]

Safety

A primary concern for patients and physicians with any treatment is safety. This concern is particularly heightened with AIT, as anaphylaxis and death have occurred with SCIT. Systemic reactions (SRs), such as urticaria, wheezing, and anaphylaxis, occur in 0.06% to 0.9% of patients undergoing SCIT.[2] There is 1 death per 2.5 million injections of SCIT.[10]

The SLIT safety profile is much higher compared with SCIT. No deaths have occurred with SLIT and SRs are less common, occurring in 0.056% of patients.[2,13,15–17,20,22] Anaphylaxis rarely occurs with SLIT. Before initiation of therapy, many practitioners prescribe an epinephrine autoinjector. Education on anaphylaxis symptoms and epinephrine autoinjector use must be provided. The first dose of SLIT is administered in the physician's office and the patient is observed for SRs.

Local reactions, such as pruritus and/or oral cavity edema, are common with SLIT. These local reactions are typically minor, nondistressing, self-limited, and viewed by patients as an inconvenience. Rarely, they lead to cessation of treatment.[16]

SUBLINGUAL IMMUNOTHERAPY FOR ALLERGIC ASTHMA

Asthma is a chronic inflammatory disease of the airways with expiratory airflow limitation. Symptoms include wheezing, coughing, chest tightness, and shortness of breath. The most common asthma phenotype is AA, with symptoms triggered by allergen

Table 3
Prescribing information for Food and Drug Administration–approved sublingual immunotherapy tablets for allergic rhinitis

Medication	Indications		Contraindications	Notes
Grastek[26]	• Allergic rhinitis • Documented allergy with positive skin testing	5–65 y	• Severe, unstable, or uncontrolled asthma	Also indicated for pollens cross-reactive with Timothy Grass
Odactra[27]	OR Specific immunoglobulin E antibodies to allergen contained in tablet	18–65 y	• History of severe local/systemic reaction to sublingual immunotherapy	Approved by the Food and Drug Administration, March 2017
Oralair[28]		10–65 y	• Eosinophilic esophagitis • Hypersensitivity to inactive ingredients in tablets	Requires 2-step escalation in children
Ragwitek[29]		18–65 y		

exposure. AA often presents in childhood and is associated with personal or family history of eczema, AR, or food allergy.[5] Eight percent of adults and 9% of children in the United States have asthma; approximately 300 million people worldwide have the disease.[31]

Indications and Contraindications

The 2017 update of the Global Strategy for Asthma Management and Prevention by the Global Initiative for Asthma now recommends consideration of SLIT in adults with AA, AR, and house dust mite (HDM) sensitivity who have asthma exacerbations despite inhaled corticosteroid treatment. These patients should have a forced expiratory volume in 1 second (FEV_1) that is 80% of predicted or better.[5] The American Academy of Allergy, Asthma and Immunology has broader indications for the use of AIT in AA (**Box 1**).[10]

Indications and contraindications when considering appropriate candidates for SLIT for AA are similar to those for AR (see **Table 1**). The contraindication regarding poorly controlled asthma is particularly important in this population, as patients with severe or uncontrolled asthma undergoing SCIT have an increased risk of SRs and death during anaphylaxis.[10]

Efficacy

Several meta-analyses and systematic reviews of SLIT for the treatment of AA have been performed (**Table 4**).[32-35] Three of these articles report a statistically significant reduction in asthma symptoms.[32-34] There was, however, a considerable degree of heterogeneity among studies. A 2015 Cochrane Review included 52 studies on SLIT for AA. Unfortunately, data from these studies were determined insufficient for a robust meta-analysis and did not report findings for areas of clinical interest such as exacerbation prevalence, quality of life, asthma symptoms, and medication use.[35]

New studies of SLIT efficacy for AA not included in these meta-analyses are now being released. The MITRA trial, a DBRCT with 834 European participants, investigated the efficacy of an HDM SLIT tablet for HDM-related AA. This study showed the addition of HDM SLIT reduced the risk of moderate or severe asthma exacerbation (hazard ratio [HR] 0.69; 95% CI 0.50–0.96, $P = .03$).[36] An HDM SLIT tablet is approved for HDM-related AA and AR in 11 European countries. A 12 standardized quality (SQ)-HDM SLIT tablet (Odactra) was approved by the FDA on March 1, 2017, for

---

Box 1
American Academy of Allergy, Asthma and Immunology indications for allergy immunotherapy in patients with specific immunoglobulin E antibodies to clinically relevant antigens

Indication

Patient preference

Inadequate response to avoidance measures

Burdensome medication requirements

Adverse effects of medications

Coexisting allergic rhinitis and asthma

Possible prevention of asthma in patients with allergic rhinitis

Adapted from Cox L, Nelson H, Lockey R, et al. Allergen immunotherapy: a practice parameter third update. J Allergy Clin Immunol 2011;127(1 Suppl):S13; with permission.

Table 4
Meta-analyses and systematic reviews of the efficacy of sublingual immunotherapy for allergic asthma

Citation	Included Studies	n	Results	Conclusion
Penagos et al,[32] 2008	9	441	Symptoms: SMD −1.14 95% CI −2.10 to −0.18 P = .02 Medication use: SMD −1.63 95% CI −2.83 to −0.44 P = .007	"SLIT with standardized extracts reduces both symptom scores and rescue medication use in children with allergic asthma compared with placebo."
Compalati et al,[33] 2009	9	476	Symptoms: SMD −0.95 95% CI −1.74 to −0.15 P = .02	"Promising evidence of efficacy for SLIT in...patients suffering from AR and AA, are herein shown. These findings suggest that more data are needed, derived from large population-based high-quality studies, and corroborated by objective outcomes, mainly for AA."
Tao et al,[34] 2014	16	794	Symptoms: SMD −0.74 95% CI −1.26 to −0.22 P = .006 Medication use: SMD −0.78 95% CI −1.45 to −0.11 P = .02	"SLIT is safe and clinically effective in reducing symptoms and medication use for allergic asthma."
Normansell et al,[35] 2015	52	5077	"[W]e were able to perform a very limited meta-analysis...Use of largely unvalidated symptom and medication scores also impeded quantitative synthesis of findings."	"This finding supports continued use of SLIT for people with other respiratory allergies, such as allergic rhinitis, who may also have well-controlled mild to moderate asthma."

Abbreviations: AA, allergic asthma; AR, allergic rhinitis; CI, confidence interval; SLIT, sublingual immunotherapy; SMD, standardized mean difference.

the treatment of HDM-associated AR, but it has not been approved for use in AA in the United States.

Durability

Studies of the efficacy of SLIT for the treatment of AA are continuing. As such, there are limited studies of the long-term durability of this treatment. One open, parallel group trial of HDM SLIT for 4 to 5 years versus standard therapy in children (n = 60) has been published.[37] This study found significant reductions in asthma diagnoses at the end of SLIT therapy. These reductions persisted for 5 years after the cessation of therapy (8.5% vs 96%, $P = .001$). Additionally, patients who underwent SLIT had a higher peak expiratory flow rate 5 years after the cessation of therapy versus controls. Although this study further supports the use of SLIT for AA, additional randomized controlled trials are needed to further evaluate the durability of the therapy.

Safety

Like SLIT for AR, SLIT for AA has a high safety profile. The previously mentioned Cochrane review analyzed results from 22 studies with 2560 patients and found, "no more than one in 100 [patients] are likely to suffer [a severe adverse event] as a result of treatment with SLIT (risk difference [RD] 0.0012, 95% CI −0.0077–0.0102; moderate-quality evidence)."[38]

The primary safety concern in SLIT for the treatment of AA is the potential to induce bronchospasm and hypoxia. Appropriate selection of patients with partly controlled asthma is the solution; that is, patients may have asthma exacerbations and symptoms but their asthma is not considered uncontrolled. The 7-item Asthma Control Questionnaire (ACQ) can be used in adults and children to identify patients with partly controlled asthma.[5] Patients respond on a 7-point scale, and the overall score is the mean of the responses (0, totally controlled; 6, severely uncontrolled). Patients who score between 1.0 and 1.5 on the ACQ are partly controlled.[39]

One of the ACQ's 7 items is the FEV_1. Even if the ACQ is not used, patients with AA being considered for SLIT should undergo pulmonary function testing. SLIT should not be initiated in patients with an FEV_1 less than 70% of predicted, as this indicates poor control. In summary, patients with partly controlled asthma, defined as an ACQ of between 1.0 and 1.5 (or other measure of control) and an FEV_1 greater than or equal to 70% of predicted may be considered possible candidates for SLIT.[5]

SUBLINGUAL IMMUNOTHERAPY FOR ATOPIC DERMATITIS

Patients with AR and AA often present with other allergic disorders. AD, sometimes referred to as eczema or atopic eczema, is a chronic inflammatory condition that often begins as a skin rash and progress to skin redness, drying, scaling, and itching. It most frequently presents in infants and children. It can persist into adulthood, or can less commonly begin in adulthood. SLIT as a possible treatment for AD has been investigated, but results are inconclusive.

A 2011 study randomized patients with HDM-related AD to receive pharmacotherapy plus HDM SLIT drops or pharmacotherapy alone. Treatment was considered effective if a subject's Severity Scoring of Atopic Dermatitis index decreased by 60% or more. Effectiveness in the SLIT group was 77.78% versus 53.85% for controls ($\chi^2 = 12.73$, $P<.05$). Daily medication use score was lower in the treatment group at 6 and 12 months as compared with the control group ($P<.01$).[40] However, a Cochrane review of AIT (4 SLIT trials, 6 SCIT trials) for the treatment of AD (733 participants) found limited, low-quality evidence that AIT is effective for AD treatment. Additional trials using high-quality allergens, patient-reported outcome measures, and low-bias study design are needed to further investigate SLIT for AD.[41]

SUBLINGUAL IMMUNOTHERAPY FOR FOOD ALLERGY

IgE-mediated food allergies often present as urticaria, vomiting, wheezing, or anaphylaxis following ingestion of an allergen-containing product. The prevalence of food allergies is increasing, as is their severity.[42] The leading food allergen resulting in anaphylaxis and death is peanut. In the past decade, the prevalence of peanut allergy has doubled in Western countries to between 1.4% and 3%.[43] AIT for food allergy is being studied as a potential treatment.

A 2017 systematic review and meta-analysis of AIT for food allergy found it "effective in raising the threshold of reactivity to a range of foods in children with IgE-mediated food allergy...."[42] Although most included studies used oral immunotherapy, 4 RCTs using SLIT were included (**Table 5**).[44–47] Pooled results revealed SLIT as effective for the treatment of food allergy (risk ratio [RR] 0.26, 95% CI 0.10–0.64, $P<.004$).

Based on these limited controlled studies, SLIT for food allergy appears to be safe in the populations tested. SRs were rare. Three of the 4 studies had no episodes of anaphylaxis requiring the use of epinephrine.[44,45,47] One patient in the study by Fleischer and colleagues[46] experienced anaphylaxis requiring treatment with epinephrine. Between 0.2% and 2.9% of SLIT doses required treatment with oral antihistamines.[44,46]

Table 5
Randomized controlled trials of the efficacy of SLIT for food allergy

Citation	n	Allergen	Results	Conclusion
Enrique et al,[44] 2005	23	Hazelnut	Change in mean quantity provoking objective symptoms: 2.29 g to 11.56 g, $P = .02$	"Our data confirm significant increases in tolerance to hazelnut after sublingual immunotherapy as assessed by double-blind, placebo-controlled food challenge, and good tolerance to this treatment."
Fernández-Rivas et al,[45] 2009	56	Peach	Change in dose needed to induce a local reaction: 9x higher Change in dose needed to induce a systemic reaction: 3x higher	"SLIT for peach allergy seems to be a promising therapeutic option that could modify the clinical reactivity of the patients to peach intake and the underlying immunologic response with a good tolerance."
Kim et al,[47] 2011	18	Peanut	The treatment group safely ingested 20 times more peanut protein than the placebo group (median 1710 vs 85 mg, $P = .011$)	"Peanut SLIT is able to safely induce clinical desensitization in children with peanut allergy, with evidence of immunologic changes suggesting a significant change in the allergic response."
Fleischer et al,[46] 2013	40	Peanut	SCD increased from 3.5 to 496 mg (median) after 44 wk. After 68 wk, median SCD increased to 996 mg.	"Peanut SLIT safely induced a modest level of desensitization in a majority of subjects compared with placebo. Longer duration of therapy showed statistically significant increases in the SCD."

Abbreviations: SCD, successfully consumed dose; SLIT, sublingual immunotherapy.

Specific indications and durability data regarding SLIT for the treatment of food allergy are lacking, however. Additional studies with larger treatment groups and longer follow-up are needed to further standardize and evaluate this therapy.

PRACTICAL APPLICATIONS OF SUBLINGUAL IMMUNOTHERAPY IN CLINICAL PRACTICE
Allergy Testing

Skin testing is one option for allergy testing and can be used provided the patient does not have contraindications (ie, use of medications that interfere with testing [**Table 6**]), beta-blocker use, uncontrolled asthma, or dermatographism. Leukotriene receptor antagonists, selective serotonin reuptake inhibitors, proton pump inhibitors, and angiotensin-converting enzyme inhibitors do not impact skin testing.[48]

Allergy skin testing may be performed via skin prick, intradermal dilution testing (IDT), and modified quantitative testing (MQT) also known as blended testing. IDT and MQT provide quantitative endpoints. Skin prick testing is a more qualitative method. Quantitative testing is not necessary if the patient knows that he or she will choose SLIT, as short escalation periods (nor no escalation) are used. In vitro laboratory testing for quantitative assessment of specific IgE is another option for allergy testing. The allergy testing panel is commonly made up of 10 to 30 antigens, with selection based on frequently encountered allergens in the local environment as well as individual medical history.

Dosing

There is significant confusion regarding dosing with immunotherapy. Contributing to this confusion is the variety of proprietary dosing units used by manufacturers, such as bioequivalent allergy units, allergy units, and SQ units. Micrograms of major allergen is the most reliable method of reporting the antigen content in an SLIT dose and should be identified when reviewing literature, if reported by the investigators. Except for antigens included in FDA-approved SLIT tablets, the optimal dose for many SLIT antigens has not been precisely identified. In general, however, total monthly maintenance doses of SLIT are a mean 87 times (median 49 times) higher than monthly SCIT maintenance doses.[18] Pediatric SLIT doses are generally equivalent to adult SLIT doses. The maximum tolerated dose, however, may be lower for younger or smaller children.[49]

Table 6
Medications that inhibit skin-based allergy testing

Medication	Maximum Days of Testing Suppression
1st-generation antihistamines	5
2nd-generation antihistamines	7
Antihistamine nasal sprays	1
Antihistamine eye drops	1
Tricyclic antidepressants	14
Benzodiazepines	7
Histamine-2 antihistamines (H_2 blockers)	2
Topical corticosteroids (at testing site)	21

Data from AAOA Clinical Care Statement Workgroup. Compendium of Clinical Care Statements. AAOA Today, 2015. Available at http://www.aaoaf.org/PDF/Clinical%20Statements/2015%20Clinical%20Care%20Statements%20Medicines%20to%20Avoid%20Before%20Allergy%20Skin%20Testing.pdf.

Most randomized controlled trials of SLIT study a single antigen. Additionally, most large-scale SLIT studies were performed in Europe, where single-antigen AIT dosing is more common. In the United States, however, the mean number of antigens used for AIT is 10.[14] Current data are limited as to the efficacy of multiantigen versus single-antigen SLIT, although this practice is commonly used in the United States.

Additional Considerations

Dosing and escalation protocols for SLIT vary widely. However, common themes are as follows: (1) SLIT dose is higher than SCIT dose, and (2) SLIT escalation is shorter than SCIT escalation. In some cases (ie, SLIT tablet dosing for adults), no escalation is used. The use of aqueous antigens is not currently approved by the FDA for SLIT application; use is off-label. If aqueous SLIT is used, the off-label nature of the treatment should be discussed with patients. Obtaining written informed consent for AIT is advocated, following a thorough discussion of the risks, benefits, and alternatives.

Following administration of the first dose in the clinician's office, SLIT is typically dosed at home. Thus, meticulous patient education is key. Patients should undergo thorough training regarding the appropriate method of taking SLIT doses, common side effects, and worrisome signs of systemic reaction or anaphylaxis. If an epinephrine autoinjector has been prescribed, patients (along with a family member or close friend) should be thoroughly educated on its use. Routine clinic follow-up to assess SLIT progress, symptom control, allergy medication use, and adherence to therapy is paramount.

Similar to SCIT, the allergy practitioner should be comfortable with his or her knowledge of SLIT before initiating this therapy in practice. Adding SLIT to a practice with no current allergy services or adding SLIT to an established SCIT practice requires planning, organization, and further study. With these considerations in mind, SLIT is a rewarding service for the provision of AIT.

SUMMARY

SLIT is effective for the treatment of AR and AA in adults and children, leading to significant reductions in symptoms and medication requirements. The effect of SLIT for AR is durable, with one study showing 8 years of benefit following a 4-year course of SLIT. The risk of moderate or severe exacerbations of AA is reduced with SLIT. Indications for SLIT use in AR have been published by the American Academy of Otolaryngology–Head and Neck Surgery and the World Health Organization. The Global Initiative for Asthma now includes SLIT in its stepwise approach to asthma treatment. A limited number of studies has shown that SLIT may have promise for the treatment of food allergy. SLIT has not, however, been demonstrated as effective for the treatment of AD based on current literature. SLIT has a higher safety profile as compared with SCIT. Although no deaths have occurred with SLIT, anaphylaxis rarely occurs. Appropriate patient selection, meticulous patient education, and routine follow-up are key for successful SLIT administration.

REFERENCES

1. Emanuel IA, Parker MJ, Traub O. Undertreatment of allergy: exploring the utility of sublingual immunotherapy. Otolaryngol Head Neck Surg 2009;140(5):615–21.
2. Seidman MD, Gurgel RK, Lin SY, et al. Clinical practice guideline: allergic rhinitis. Otolaryngol Head Neck Surg 2015;152(1 Suppl):S1–43.
3. Meltzer EO, Bukstein DA. The economic impact of allergic rhinitis and current guidelines for treatment. Ann Allergy Asthma Immunol 2011;106(2 Suppl):S12–6.

4. Loftus PA, Wise SK. Epidemiology and economic burden of asthma. Int Forum Allergy Rhinol 2015;5(Suppl 1):S7–10.
5. Global Initiative for Asthma. Global strategy for asthma management and prevention, 2017. Available at: www.ginasthma.org.
6. Bloomfield SF, Rook GA, Scott EA, et al. Time to abandon the hygiene hypothesis: new perspectives on allergic disease, the human microbiome, infectious disease prevention and the role of targeted hygiene. Perspect Public Health 2016;136(4): 213–24.
7. Liu AH. Revisiting the hygiene hypothesis for allergy and asthma. J Allergy Clin Immunol 2015;136(4):860–5.
8. Mattos JL, Woodard CR, Payne SC. Trends in common rhinologic illnesses: analysis of U.S. healthcare surveys 1995-2007. Int Forum Allergy Rhinol 2011;1(1): 3–12.
9. Maurer M, Zuberbier T. Undertreatment of rhinitis symptoms in Europe: findings from a cross-sectional questionnaire survey. Allergy 2007;62(9):1057–63.
10. Cox L, Nelson H, Lockey R, et al. Allergen immunotherapy: a practice parameter, third update. J Allergy Clin Immunol 2011;127(1 Suppl):S1–55.
11. Curtis H. The immunizing cure of hayfever. Med News 1900;77:16–8.
12. CSM update: desensitising vaccines. Br Med J (Clin Res Ed) 1986;293(6552): 948.
13. Bousquet J, Khaltaev N, Cruz AA, et al. Allergic rhinitis and its impact on asthma (ARIA) 2008 update (in collaboration with the World Health Organization, GA(2) LEN and AllerGen). Allergy 2008;63(Suppl 86):8–160.
14. Wise SK, Schlosser RJ. Evidence-based practice: sublingual immunotherapy for allergic rhinitis. Otolaryngol Clin North Am 2012;45(5):1045–54.
15. Jutel M, Agache I, Bonini S, et al. International consensus on allergy immunotherapy. J Allergy Clin Immunol 2015;136(3):556–68.
16. Radulovic S, Calderon MA, Wilson D, et al. Sublingual immunotherapy for allergic rhinitis. Cochrane Database Syst Rev 2010;(12):CD002893.
17. Lin SY, Erekosima N, Kim JM, et al. Sublingual immunotherapy for the treatment of allergic rhinoconjunctivitis and asthma: a systematic review. JAMA 2013;309(12): 1278–88.
18. Cox LS, Larenas Linnemann D, Nolte H, et al. Sublingual immunotherapy: a comprehensive review. J Allergy Clin Immunol 2006;117(5):1021–35.
19. Shaikh WA, Shaikh SW. A prospective study on the safety of sublingual immunotherapy in pregnancy. Allergy 2012;67(6):741–3.
20. Kim JM, Lin SY, Suarez-Cuervo C, et al. Allergen-specific immunotherapy for pediatric asthma and rhinoconjunctivitis: a systematic review. Pediatrics 2013; 131(6):1155–67.
21. Devillier P, Dreyfus JF, Demoly P, et al. A meta-analysis of sublingual allergen immunotherapy and pharmacotherapy in pollen-induced seasonal allergic rhinoconjunctivitis. BMC Med 2014;12:71.
22. Di Bona D, Plaia A, Leto-Barone MS, et al. Efficacy of grass pollen allergen sublingual immunotherapy tablets for seasonal allergic rhinoconjunctivitis: a systematic review and meta-analysis. JAMA Intern Med 2015;175(8):1301–9.
23. Marogna M, Tomassetti D, Bernasconi A, et al. Preventive effects of sublingual immunotherapy in childhood: an open randomized controlled study. Ann Allergy Asthma Immunol 2008;101(2):206–11.
24. Novembre E, Galli E, Landi F, et al. Coseasonal sublingual immunotherapy reduces the development of asthma in children with allergic rhinoconjunctivitis. J Allergy Clin Immunol 2004;114(4):851–7.

25. La Rosa M, Ranno C, Andre C, et al. Double-blind placebo-controlled evaluation of sublingual-swallow immunotherapy with standardized *Parietaria judaica* extract in children with allergic rhinoconjunctivitis. J Allergy Clin Immunol 1999; 104(2 Pt 1):425–32.

26. Timothy grass pollen allergen extract [package insert]. Merck Sharp & Dohme Corp., Kenilworth, NJ; April 2014. Available at: https://www.fda.gov/downloads/BiologicsBloodVaccines/Allergenics/UCM393184.pdf. Accessed April 18, 2017.

27. House dust mite (*Dermatophagoides farinae* and *Dermatophagoides pteronyssinus*) allergen extract tablet for sublingual use [package insert]. Kenilworth, NJ: Merck Sharp & Dohme Corp; 2017. Available at: https://www.fda.gov/downloads/BiologicsBloodVaccines/Allergenics/UCM544382.pdf. Accessed April 18, 2017.

28. Sweet Vernal, Orchard, Perennial Rye, Timothy, and Kentucky blue grass mixed pollens allergen extract [package insert]. Stallergenes S.A., Antony, France; 2014. Available at: https://www.fda.gov/downloads/BiologicsBloodVaccines/Allergenics/UCM391580.pdf. Accessed April 18, 2017.

29. Short ragweed pollen allergen extract [package insert]. Kenilworth, NJ: Merck Sharp & Dohme Corp; 2014. Available at: https://www.fda.gov/downloads/BiologicsBloodVaccines/Allergenics/UCM393600.pdf. Accessed April 18, 2017.

30. Marogna M, Spadolini I, Massolo A, et al. Long-lasting effects of sublingual immunotherapy according to its duration: a 15-year prospective study. J Allergy Clin Immunol 2010;126(5):969–75.

31. Mener DJ, Lin SY. Improvement and prevention of asthma with concomitant treatment of allergic rhinitis and allergen-specific therapy. Int Forum Allergy Rhinol 2015;5(Suppl 1):S45–50.

32. Penagos M, Passalacqua G, Compalati E, et al. Metaanalysis of the efficacy of sublingual immunotherapy in the treatment of allergic asthma in pediatric patients, 3 to 18 years of age. Chest 2008;133(3):599–609.

33. Compalati E, Passalacqua G, Bonini M, et al. The efficacy of sublingual immunotherapy for house dust mites respiratory allergy: results of a GA2LEN meta-analysis. Allergy 2009;64(11):1570–9.

34. Tao L, Shi B, Shi G, et al. Efficacy of sublingual immunotherapy for allergic asthma: retrospective meta-analysis of randomized, double-blind and placebo-controlled trials. Clin Respir J 2014;8(2):192–205.

35. Normansell R, Kew KM, Bridgman AL. Sublingual immunotherapy for asthma. Cochrane Database Syst Rev 2015;(8):CD011293.

36. Virchow JC, Backer V, Kuna P, et al. Efficacy of a house dust mite sublingual allergen immunotherapy tablet in adults with allergic asthma: a randomized clinical trial. JAMA 2016;315(16):1715–25.

37. Di Rienzo V, Marcucci F, Puccinelli P, et al. Long-lasting effect of sublingual immunotherapy in children with asthma due to house dust mite: a 10-year prospective study. Clin Exp Allergy 2003;33(2):206–10.

38. Mosbech H, Deckelmann R, de Blay F, et al. Standardized quality (SQ) house dust mite sublingual immunotherapy tablet (ALK) reduces inhaled corticosteroid use while maintaining asthma control: a randomized, double-blind, placebo-controlled trial. J Allergy Clin Immunol 2014;134(3):568–75.e7.

39. Juniper EF, Bousquet J, Abetz L, et al. Identifying 'well-controlled' and 'not well-controlled' asthma using the asthma control questionnaire. Respir Med 2006; 100(4):616–21.

40. Qin YE, Mao JR, Sang YC, et al. Clinical efficacy and compliance of sublingual immunotherapy with *Dermatophagoides farinae* drops in patients with atopic dermatitis. Int J Dermatol 2014;53(5):650–5.

41. Tam H, Calderon MA, Manikam L, et al. Specific allergen immunotherapy for the treatment of atopic eczema. Cochrane Database Syst Rev 2016;(2):CD008774.

42. Nurmatov U, Dhami S, Arasi S, et al. Allergen immunotherapy for IgE-mediated food allergy: a systematic review and meta-analysis. Allergy 2017;72(8):1133–47.

43. Du Toit G, Roberts G, Sayre PH, et al. Randomized trial of peanut consumption in infants at risk for peanut allergy. N Engl J Med 2015;372(9):803–13.

44. Enrique E, Pineda F, Malek T, et al. Sublingual immunotherapy for hazelnut food allergy: a randomized, double-blind, placebo-controlled study with a standardized hazelnut extract. J Allergy Clin Immunol 2005;116(5):1073–9.

45. Fernández-Rivas M, Garrido Fernandez S, Nadal JA, et al. Randomized double-blind, placebo-controlled trial of sublingual immunotherapy with a Pru p 3 quantified peach extract. Allergy 2009;64(6):876–83.

46. Fleischer DM, Burks AW, Vickery BP, et al. Sublingual immunotherapy for peanut allergy: a randomized, double-blind, placebo-controlled multicenter trial. J Allergy Clin Immunol 2013;131(1):119–27.e1–7.

47. Kim EH, Bird JA, Kulis M, et al. Sublingual immunotherapy for peanut allergy: clinical and immunologic evidence of desensitization. J Allergy Clin Immunol 2011;127(3):640–6.e1.

48. AAOA clinical care statement workgroup. Compendium of clinical care statements. AAOA today. 2015. Available at: http://www.aaoaf.org/PDF/2015.Clinical Care Statements Bro.web.pdf. Accessed April 24, 2017.

49. Larenas-Linnemann D. Subcutaneous and sublingual immunotherapy in children: complete update on controversies, dosing, and efficacy. Curr Allergy Asthma Rep 2008;8(6):465–74.

Contemporary Pharmacotherapy for Allergic Rhinitis and Chronic Rhinosinusitis

Saied Ghadersohi, MD, Bruce K. Tan, MD, MS*

KEYWORDS

- Chronic rhinosinusitis (CRS) • Type 2 inflammation • Novel pharmacotherapy
- Biologics • Immune specific targeting

KEY POINTS

- Chronic rhinosinusitis (CRS) is driven by chronic inflammation of the sinonasal mucosa initiated by undefined factors. In contrast, allergic rhinitis (AR) causes nasal inflammation following nasal exposure to sensitized environmental allergens.
- A type 2 inflammatory response with interleukin (IL)C2 cells, Th2 cells, eosinophils, basophils and mast cells along with the cytokines IL-4, IL-5 and IL-13 dominates CRS with nasal polyposis and a substantial fraction of patients with CRS without nasal polyps.
- New biologics indicated for asthma have been studied in randomized controlled trials of patients with AR and CRS, and demonstrate efficacy largely in a "salvage" setting.

INTRODUCTION

Chronic rhinosinusitis (CRS) is an inflammatory disease of the nasal airways and paranasal sinuses. The condition is defined by more than 12 weeks of nasal obstruction, nasal discharge, facial pain/pressure, and reduced/lost smell, combined with either computed tomography (CT) or endoscopic examination with evidence of inflammation, polyps, or purulence.[1,2] In population-based surveys of European and US populations, between 10.9% and 11.9% of respondents had CRS-appropriate symptoms, although the percentage of these with CT or endoscopic evidence of inflammation remains undefined.[3,4] The most recent consensus statements both from US and European authorities posit that current evidence suggests CRS is a chronic inflammatory process mediated by a complex interplay of environmental and genetic factors that are not fully elucidated.[1,2]

Disclosures: Nothing to disclose.
Department of Otolaryngology–Head and Neck Surgery, Northwestern University, Feinberg School of Medicine, 676 North Saint Clair Suite #1325, Chicago, IL 60611, USA
* Corresponding author.
E-mail address: btan@nm.org

Otolaryngol Clin N Am 50 (2017) 1135–1151
http://dx.doi.org/10.1016/j.otc.2017.08.009
0030-6665/17/© 2017 Elsevier Inc. All rights reserved.

CRS is commonly further classified into 2 subsets based on its clinical phenotype: those with polyps (CRSwNP) and those without (CRSsNP). The CRSsNP subgroup exhibits a wide variation in symptomatic and objective manifestations, but those with CRSwNP typically have more severe radiographic disease that can be resistant to conventional medical and surgical therapeutic measures. Although convenient, this classification has proven overly simplistic because it does not fully reflect the disease course. For example, there is a subset of CRSwNP patients who have aspirin-exacerbated respiratory disease (AERD), which is well recognized to be frequently recalcitrant to medical and surgical treatments.[5–8] To define pathobiologically coherent disease subtypes in CRS, there has been an evolution from subtyping using clinical characteristics (eg, presence of polyps, atopy, or asthma) to one based on the specific immunologic pathways driving the disease.[9–11]

Allergic rhinitis (AR) is similarly an inflammatory disorder characterized by symptoms of rhinitis, including rhinorrhea, blockage, sneezing, or itching following exposure to an environmental allergen to which the patient is sensitized. Typical allergens include dust mites; grass, tree, or weed pollens; cats; dogs; and molds,[12,13] and hypersensitivity is detected by skin or serum testing. AR has a significant effect on patient quality of life (QoL); additionally it is often comorbid to and contributes to the development and progression of asthma.[12] Although prior studies demonstrate that patients with CRS do have an elevated prevalence of AR, AR is far from universal among patients with CRS.[14,15] Furthermore, exposure studies demonstrate that the changes in the sinuses following allergen exposure are relatively mild compared with those observed in CRS.[16]

INFLAMMATORY PATHWAYS IN CHRONIC RHINOSINUSITIS AND ALLERGIC RHINITIS

In Western countries, CRSwNP has been associated with type 2 inflammatory responses characterized by eosinophils, mast cells, and basophils, elevated total immunoglobulin (Ig)E and cytokines, including interleukin (IL)-5, IL-4, and IL-13.[9,11,17–19] Classically, the initiation of type 2 inflammation was postulated to begin with allergen/antigen uptake by dendritic cells that processed the antigens and influenced the T-cell response through the production of cytokines, including IL-4, that differentiated Th0 cells into Th2 lymphocytes.[20–23] More recently, epithelial cells have been shown to have innate responses that can directly activate a class of lymphocytes called innate lymphoid cells that produce many of the same cytokines traditionally ascribed to T cells. For example, epithelial exposure to irritants, and antigens induces epithelial production of one or a combination of these initiators, IL-25, IL-33, and Thymic stromal lymphopoietin (TSLP) that can directly activate innate lymphoid 2 cells (ILC2 cells) that produce the key pathogenic type 2 cytokines IL-5, IL-13, and to a lesser extent IL-4.[20–25] IL-5 primarily facilitates differentiation, migration, activation, and survival of eosinophils, B cells, and basophils.[26,27] IL-13, which shares a common receptor with IL-4, is thought to have larger effects on structural cells causing epithelial cells to produce mucus and smooth muscle hyperreactivity.[28] IL-4 influences cells of the adaptive immune system driving Th0 to Th2 cell differentiation and B-cell isotype switching and the production and secretion of antibodies. Of these factors, IL-5, IL-13, and the initiator TSLP have consistently been demonstrated to be elevated in CRSwNP nasal tissue, whereas elevated IL-4, IL-33, and IL-25 have less consistent data in the CRSwNP patient population.[29,30] However, this pattern may further vary with ethnicity or geography, because more than half of Chinese patients are noted to have a noneosinophilic inflammation.[11,17,31] We recommend referencing a recent review by Schleimer[32] for an excellent review of type 2 inflammation in CRSwNP.

Although CRSsNP was traditionally described as a type 1 inflammatory response with elevated neutrophils and lower levels of eosinophils, this view has been challenged by 2 recent publications that find that it is a heterogeneous inflammatory response with type 1, 2, and 3 responses.[1,10,11,17] These studies also demonstrate that in Western countries, approximately 30% to 50% of patients with CRSsNP have elevated markers of type 2 inflammation, similar to CRSwNP, making this the most common endotype found in CRSsNP. There were also minor but significant subsets of patients with CRSsNP that had elevated IL-17 (4%–25%) and interferon-γ (6%–21%) in their nasal mucosa.[1,10,18] Clearly further research is still needed to understand the interplay of these pathways with correlations to disease phenotypes, treatment responsiveness, and prognosis.

Although many of the same type 2 mediators, effector cells, and cytokines found in CRS are also found in AR, a fundamental difference is AR is triggered by an IgE-dependent mast cell degranulation due to exposure to a specific antigen that the patient has a previously developed systemic atopic hypersensitivity.[33] In the late phase following allergen exposure, recruitment of other effector cells, including eosinophils and Th2 cells, can be found.[13,34] However, atopy does not significantly influence symptom severity, extent of sinus disease on CT scans, and likelihood of undergoing revision surgery among patients with CRS.[35]

CONVENTIONAL CHRONIC RHINOSINUSITIS AND ALLERGIC RHINITIS TREATMENT

The controversy over the pathologic underpinnings of CRS led to significant variability in how CRS is cared for medically. Currently, intranasal saline irrigations, topical intranasal steroids, oral steroids, and surgical management when medical therapy fails represent contemporary care options for which evidence of efficacy exists.[1,2] Topical saline irrigations have been shown to reduce symptom scores when used as sole agents or adjuncts to intranasal steroids.[36] The efficacy of topical intranasal steroids has been substantiated in randomized clinical trials (RCTs) in AR and meta-analysis of RCTs of CRSsNP and CRSwNP with evidence for modest improvements in symptom outcome scores, and polyp size reduction, especially in those who had previously undergone surgery.[37–42] Short courses of systemic steroids have also been well studied in CRSwNP, showing improvements in polyp size, symptoms, and outcomes.[43–45] There is no high-level evidence supporting the use of systemic steroids in CRSsNP, although they are likely to be effective in the subset of patients who have elevated type 2 inflammation.[46] Despite almost universal prescription for CRS care, strong evidence for the efficacy of antibiotics is still lacking. Overall, recent consensus statements indicate against or insufficient evidence for nonmacrolide oral antibiotics.[1,2] Additionally, long-term macrolide therapy that has been studied in 2 randomized, placebo-controlled studies drew mixed conclusions, with one study showing a benefit and another with no benefit likely due to differential recruitment of CRSwNP and postsurgical patients in the 2 studies.[47–49]

The use of intranasal and oral second-generation antihistamines remains first-line therapy for intermittent AR but not in CRS.[34,50] In CRS, leukotriene inhibitors have a slight inferiority as a single modality to prevent nasal polyp recurrence compared with other agents, such as intranasal steroids.[51,52] In AR, leukotriene inhibitors are also inferior in symptom control compared with intranasal steroids and antihistamines; however, these agents could be considered for dual therapy of patients with persistent asthma.[50] Therefore, current recommendations are against routine use of leukotriene inhibitors for CRS and AR as first-line agents.[1,2,50]

Studies in patients with AR show that proper implementation of ARIA (allergic rhinitis and its impact on asthma) guidelines can result in symptom control in 80% to 90% of patients.[53,54] By contrast, despite implementation of "appropriate medical therapy," rates of symptomatic improvement are modest and variable (38%–51%) in CRS depending on the threshold of success, symptom domain, and duration of follow-up.[17,55,56] Patients with CRS failing appropriate medical therapy are offered endoscopic sinus surgery that has been shown in prospective observational studies to deliver significantly increased QoL compared with continued medical management.[57,58] In fact, emerging evidence suggests earlier surgical intervention may prevent the development of adult-onset asthma.[58,59] However, there still remain recalcitrant patients in high-risk groups, particularly those with nasal polyps (AERD, eosinophilic mucin, comorbid asthma) who either do not respond to medical or surgical interventions or have comorbidities for which these interventions are contraindicated.

Thus, unlike other atopic airway diseases like asthma or AR, CRS uniquely has a minimally invasive surgical management option with demonstrated efficacy. Thus, when considering the role of pharmacotherapy in CRS, we propose that evidence for its efficacy may increasingly be judged on the basis of its intended purpose and temporal association with surgery. This nomenclature is well developed in oncology, where both medical and surgical treatments are critical to the standard of care, but have, to our knowledge, not been applied in CRS care. Thus, "induction" pharmacotherapy may be used to induce a remission of CRS without surgery, "adjuvant" pharmacotherapy may be applied around the time of surgery to enhance the chance of remission, "maintenance" pharmacotherapy may be used to sustain a remission, and "salvage" pharmacotherapy may be applied when conventional medical and surgical options have failed. Although many prior pharmacotherapy studies of CRS were used for induction, the more recent "biologics" have been studied in CRS largely in the context of salvage treatment for CRSwNP (**Fig. 1, Table 1**).

BIOLOGIC THERAPY IN CHRONIC RHINOSINUSITIS
Interleukin-5 Pathway

Reslizumab
The earliest RCT using biologics was published in 2006 using reslizumab (humanized anti-IL-5) for patients with CRSwNP with bilateral grade 3 or 4 nasal polyps or recurrent nasal polyps after surgery. This agent was approved by the Food and Drug Administration (FDA) in 2016 for add-on maintenance treatment of severe eosinophilic

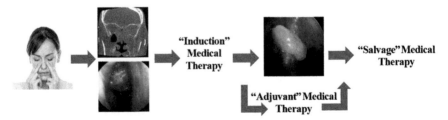

Fig. 1. Roles for biologic therapy in the treatment of CRS. "Induction" medical therapy: could be combined with appropriate medical therapy, fewer complications than surgery, and at least as efficacious. "Adjuvant" medical therapy enhances effects and durability of surgery. "Salvage" medical therapy: reduces the need for revision surgery, reserved for patients with recalcitrant disease.

asthma. IL-5 has been found to be elevated in nasal polyp tissue compared with healthy controls, with the highest concentrations in patients with comorbid nonallergic asthma or AERD.[60,61] A total of 24 patients were enrolled and divided to receive placebo, or a single 1-mg/kg or a 3-mg/kg intravenous dose. Reslizumab was well tolerated in patients, with the most common adverse event being upper respiratory tract infection symptoms. In the active treatment groups, the investigators found polyp size improved in approximately half of the patients at 4 weeks but 4 patients had deterioration in polyp scores by 12 weeks. Nasal peak inspiratory flow rates (NPIF) and symptoms were not different at any time point. Biologic activity analysis showed peripheral eosinophil counts, peripheral and local IL-5 levels, and eosinophil cationic protein (ECP) levels decreased up to the 8-week time point, but peripheral eosinophil counts rebounded to higher levels by 24 and 32 weeks. As a phase 1 trial, the study was underpowered to detect the difference in polyp size or symptoms. However, in comparing baseline characteristics of responders with nonresponders, they noted that the responders had higher baseline nasal IL-5 levels, alluding to a possible role for nasal IL-5 in predicting responders.[62]

Mepolizumab
Mepolizumab, another anti-IL-5 humanized antibody that was FDA approved for severe eosinophilic asthma in 2015, has been investigated in CRS. Twenty patients with CRSwNP (grade 3 or 4 or recurrent after surgery) were given two 750-mg doses 28 days apart and results were compared with 10 patients who were given placebo. This trial was better powered to assess the efficacy of anti-IL-5 treatment compared with the previous study of reslizumab by the same group. Sixty percent of the treated group compared with 10% of the placebo group had improvements in the primary endpoint of nasal polyp scores at 8 weeks. There were also significant improvements in the secondary endpoints of radiographic severity, blood eosinophil levels, ECP, and blood IL-5R levels at 8 weeks. Patients also noted decreased postnasal drip and better smell and congestion at 8 weeks, but rhinorrhea was unaffected. Interestingly, the responders were not noted to have elevated nasal IL-5 levels nor was a robust rebound eosinophilia noted.[63] In review of the clinical trials registry, it appears that an additional study of mepolizumab has recently completed recruitment of 105 patients with CRSwNP refractory to medical and surgical therapy with the primary endpoint being the need for surgery after treatment.[64]

Benralizumab
Another agent that could potentially have some promise for inhibiting the IL-5 pathway in CRS is benralizumab. Most recently, a 2016 phase 3 RCT in patients with refractory eosinophilic asthma showed that those treated had higher prebronchodilator forced expiratory volume in 1 second and lower annual asthma exacerbation rates.[65] This agent works by competitively inhibiting the IL-5 receptor and, due to a fucosylation of the monoclonal antibody, it more strongly binds natural killer cell receptors causing an antibody-dependent, cell-mediated cytotoxicity of effector cells, including eosinophils and basophils, which have also been implicated in CRSwNP.[27,66] Currently there is an ongoing phase 2 RCT of subcutaneous administration of benralizumab in eosinophilic chronic sinusitis that is estimated to be completed in October 2017.[67]

Immunoglobulin E Pathway

Omalizumab
Omalizumab is a humanized anti-IgE monoclonal antibody that binds free IgE, preventing binding to receptors on mast cells and basophils. Previous studies have

Table 1
Biologics studied in patients with CRS

Study	Drug Name and Mechanism	Study Population	End Points	Adverse Events	Interesting Points or Problem with Study
Randomized clinical trials					
Gevaert et al,[75] 2013	Omalizumab - Anti-IgE	24 patients - CRSwNP with comorbid asthma	1. Endoscopic nasal polyp scores 2. CT scores 3. Nasal and asthma symptom/QoL questionnaires	URI symptoms	Small sample size. Was effective independent of allergy status or elevated serum IgE.
Pinto et al,[74] 2010	Omalizumab - Anti-IgE	14 patients - 12 with CRSwNP	1. Lund Mackay Score 2. SNOT-20 3. UPSIT 4. NPIF 5. Eosinophil levels	Concern for anaphylaxis, 1 patient with malignancy	Showed minor improvements in radiographic severity. Patients resumed previous therapy and were allowed to have "rescue" medications.
Gevaert et al,[62] 2006	Reslizumab - Anti-IL-5	24 pts CRSwNP (grade 3–4 or surgical salvage)	1. Endoscopic nasal polyp scores (qualitative) 2. NPIF 3. Serum eosinophilia 4. IL-5 levels 5. ECP levels	URI symptoms	1. Increased baseline IL-5 predicted responsiveness 2. Rebound eosinophilia

Study	Drug	Population	Outcomes	Adverse events	Results
Gevaert et al,[63] 2011	Mepolizumab - Anti-IL-5	30 pts CRSwNP (grade 3–4 or surgical salvage)	1. Endoscopic nasal polyp scores 2. CT scores 3. NPIF 4. Symptoms 5. Serum eosinophilia 6. IL-5R levels 7. ECP levels	URI symptoms	1. Significantly improved symptoms and reduced nasal polyps. 2. Follow-up to 48 wk
Bachert et al,[84] 2016	Dupilumab - mAb to IL-4R-α subunit	60 CRSwNP with and without asthma	1. Endoscopic nasal polyp scores 2. CT scores 3. UPSIT 4. NPIF 5. SNOT-22 6. Serum IgE 7. IL-5 levels 8. Eotaxin-3 levels	Nasopharyngitis, HA, injection site reactions	1. Dramatic improvements in symptoms and biomarkers of type 2 inflammation.
Retrospective studies					
Vennera Mdel et al,[73] 2011	Omalizumab - Anti-IgE	18 severe asthmatic patients with nasal polyps	1. Endoscopic nasal polyp scores 2. Intranasal steroid use		
Chandra et al,[76] 2016	Omalizumab - Anti-IgE	25 patients with asthma and CRS	1. Antibiotic use, 60% reduction 2. Systemic steroid use, 42% reduction		

Abbreviations: CRS, chronic rhinosinusitis; CRSwNP, CRS with nasal polyps; CT, computed tomography; ECP, eosinophil cationic protein; Ig, immunoglobulin; IL, interleukin; NPIF, nasal peak inspiratory flow rate; SNOT, Sino-Nasal Outcome Test; UPSIT, University of Pennsylvania Smell Identification Test.

shown that this agent can also decrease IgE receptors on effector cells.[68] Omalizumab was approved for treatment of severe allergic asthma in 2003.

Of the biological agents discussed, omalizumab is the only agent that has been studied for AR treatment. In 2000, a European study randomly assigned 251 patients with seasonal AR with positive testing to birch pollen to receive omalizumab versus placebo. They noted significantly decreased serum IgE levels, improved average daily nasal symptom scores, QoL questionnaires, and decreased use of rescue antihistamines.[69] These findings were again noted in a dose-dependent fashion in a second RCT of 536 patients with ragweed-induced seasonal AR.[70] A separate RCT of 289 patients with perennial AR also noted symptomatic improvement relative to placebo.[71] Despite demonstrated efficacy, the use of omalizumab in the AR patient population remains limited to those with severe disease and comorbid severe allergic asthma due to the high cost and lack of an AR indication for this drug.[34]

Evidence for efficacy of omalizumab has been reported in case series and case reports of patients with CRSwNP with comorbid asthma. These studies showed significantly reduced endoscopic nasal polyp scores at 16 weeks and decreased intranasal steroid use from 95% to 42% at the end of follow-up.[72,73] It should be noted that omalizumab in these cases was generally applied in a "salvage" situation, as patients all had failed medical and surgical management of their CRSwNP.

The first RCT evaluating omalizumab in patients with CRS was published in 2010. Fourteen patients (12 CRSwNP and 2 CRSsNP) were randomized to receive placebo or subcutaneous omalizumab every 4 weeks for 6 months. Interestingly, the study suffered from poor recruitment, and patients were allowed to continue previous treatment regimens. Although they were similar at baseline, these factors limited the study's ability to assess efficacy of omalizumab in "induction" therapy. This study found radiographic opacification did significantly decrease from 76.1% to 60.0% before to after omalizumab treatment, but similar changes were not observed in the placebo arm. However, there was no significant difference in any of the secondary outcomes, including nasal endoscopy scores, Sino-Nasal Outcome Test (SNOT-20) scores, University of Pennsylvania Smell Identification Test (UPSIT) olfactory testing, NPIF testing, and eosinophil levels in nasal lavage. Patients in the trial were also allowed to use "rescue" medications during the trial period and it was noted that the omalizumab group needed fewer systemic steroid treatments.[74]

The second omalizumab RCT was published in 2014, whereby 24 allergic and nonallergic patients with CRSwNP and comorbid asthma were 2:1 randomized to receive 4 to 8 doses of omalizumab subcutaneously or placebo. Unlike the prior study, patients in the treatment arm were noted to have significantly decreased endoscopic nasal polyp scores and Lund Mackay CT scores. Secondary outcomes of improved asthma QoL measures and nasal symptom questionnaires were noted in the omalizumab-treated patients. Interestingly, both allergic and nonallergic patients noted significant improvement in outcomes, indicating that local IgE may play a role in mediating the inflammatory process in nonallergic patients.[75]

Last, Chandra and colleagues[76] retrospectively examined a series of 25 patients with asthma and CRS, in which 8 of the 25 had CRSwNP. They assessed the antibiotic and steroid use in patients before and after treatment with omalizumab. Their analysis specifically looked at prescriptions given for CRS or CRS with asthma exacerbations, and excluded those for asthma alone. They noted a statistically significant 60% reduction in the use of antibiotics in their series. The study also noted a nonstatistically significant 42% reduction in systemic steroid use.

Although generally safe, omalizumab is associated with some concerns about anaphylaxis, and malignancy, side effects. The anaphylaxis risk, as assessed by the omalizumab joint task force (OJTF), was 0.09%. The OJTF thus recommends an observation period in clinic after administration, and patients should be given precautions for signs and symptoms of anaphylaxis and an epinephrine autoinjector.[77–79] After a 2003 asthma omalizumab trial, there was a numerical imbalance of malignancy rates (primarily nonmelanoma skin cancers and other solid tumors) of 0.5% compared with 0.2% in the placebo group.[80] In a larger study, 7857 asthmatic subjects with 5004 omalizumab-treated patients were compared with patients not treated with omalizumab and found no difference in malignancy rates.[81] However, the cohort had poor follow-up and excluded patients with prior cancer history.[82]

Interleukin-4/13 Pathway

Dupilumab
Another studied pathway for which RCT data exist in CRS is the IL-4/13 pathway. Although previous studies evaluating antibodies against IL-4 or IL-13 have been disappointing in asthma,[83] IL-4 and IL-13 receptor share a common alpha subunit that makes blockade of the receptor an attractive target. Dupilumab is an anti-IL-4/13 alpha subunit receptor antibody that has just been approved for atopic dermatitis. In a very recent RCT, 60 patients with CRSwNP were enrolled (35 also had comorbid asthma) with a 1:1 randomization to dupilumab or placebo for 16 weeks. Patients also continued intranasal steroid therapy. They noted at least a 1-point polyp score improvement in 70% of treated patients compared with 20% in the placebo group at the 16-week endpoint, and this difference was apparent as early as the 4-week timepoint. Significant improvement was also noted in Lund-Mackay CT scores, percent maxillary sinus opacification, NPIF scores, symptom scores, SNOT-22, and UPSIT olfactory scores compared with placebo-treated patients. Decreased levels of serum total IgE levels and eotaxin-3 levels were noted in the patients receiving dupilumab. The most common side effects noted were nasopharyngitis, headache, and injection site reactions.[84]

OTHER ONGOING STUDIES IN CHRONIC RHINOSINUSITIS
Siglec-8 Targeting

Siglecs, which stands for sialic acid-binding immunoglobulinlike lectins, are a family of transmembrane glycoproteins that activate intracellular pathways.[85] Siglec-8 is specific to the surface of human eosinophils, mast cells, and basophils.[86] Binding of antibody to siglec-8 has been shown in in-vitro studies to induce apoptosis in cytokine-activated eosinophils or preventing release of mediators from mast cells.[87] This provides a unique method of inhibition of these target cells in CRS.[88] There is currently a phase 2 RCT with the drug AK001 in patients with CRSwNP.[89]

Interleukin-33 Targeting

Another epithelial-derived cytokine that has been shown to be elevated in nasal polyps at the gene expression level is IL-33.[90,91] IL-33 influences differentiation and activation of Th2 cells, ILC2 cells, mast cells, basophils, and the cytokine IL-13.[20] Results are pending from a phase 1 RCT in 41 patients with CRSwNP and healthy volunteers treated with AMG 282, a monoclonal antibody that inhibits binding of IL-33.[92]

OTHER POTENTIAL TARGETS IN CHRONIC RHINOSINUSITIS
TSLP Targeting

As discussed earlier, TSLP is a potent epithelial-derived cytokine that stimulates dendritic cell–driven Th2 polarization and ILC2 activation that is elevated in nasal polyp tissue.[21,90,93] Anti-TSLP targeting has shown promise in recent studies of patients with asthma treated with a humanized monoclonal antibody AMG-157. This study found the severity of asthma attacks and blood and sputum eosinophils decreased significantly in the AMG-157–treated arms.[94] Although there are ongoing clinical trials with AMG 157 for atopic dermatitis and asthma, there are no ongoing clinical trials in patients with CRS.

Small Molecule Inhibitors of the Type 2 Pathway

There have a been a few interesting small molecules specifically targeting Th2 pathways GATA3, CRTH2, and dexpramipexole. GATA-3 is a transcription factor that controls the differentiation of Th2 and ILC2 cells that produce IL-4, IL-13, and IL-5 (**Table 2**).[95] The GATA-3 DNAzyme was designed to penetrate cells and target the GATA-3 RNA for cleavage.[96,97] A recent phase 2 RCT of SB010 (GATA-3 DNAzyme) was used in patients with mild allergic asthma with sputum eosinophilia and showed the drug attenuates early-phase and late-phase asthmatic responses after allergen exposure. Biologically, this study noted reduced mast cell activation, airway eosinophilia, and serum IL-5 levels.[97] There have yet to be any investigations of this agent in a CRS patient population.

The CRTH2 antagonist OC000459 was studied in patients with asthma and AR and shown to block the effects of Prostaglandin D2, which contributes to accumulation and activation of Th2 cells, eosinophils, and basophils in tissues.[98–100] Last, dexpramipexole is an investigational small molecule drug used for amyotrophic lateral sclerosis that incidentally was noted to significantly decrease absolute eosinophil levels. Investigations are under way and have shown some promise in decreasing eosinophil levels in patients with CRS.[101,102]

CHALLENGES WITH BIOLOGICS

Although treatment with targeted therapy shows promise for CRS treatment, currently FDA-approved biological options are costly and do not appear to durably resolve findings or symptoms of CRS after treatment cessation. Although CRS is not directly a life-threatening disease, prior studies suggest general QoL impairment and health utility values are comparable to more serious illnesses. Our prior studies suggest that given average utility values in CRS, treatments that *cure* CRS for less than $11,000 per year would be cost-effective using a willingness to pay threshold of $50,000 per quality-adjusted life year.[103] Additionally, the efficacy of these agents has yet to be weighed against the costs and efficacy of conventional medical therapy and endoscopic sinus surgery that is efficacious in a significant fraction of patients.

Given the cost of currently approved biologics (omalizumab and mepolizumab), if cost trends continue, it is likely that biologics will be reserved for salvage therapy for patients with CRSwNP with comorbid severe asthma, AERD, or recalcitrance after sinus surgery. For biologics to gain a role for induction or maintenance therapy in CRS, it is likely novel pharmacologic agents will have to be relatively inexpensive. Other novel applications of new pharmaceuticals may be their role in an adjuvant setting to help enhance the long-term efficacy of endoscopic sinus surgery. Significantly increased investment in studies of CRS are needed to define the safety, efficacy, and role these novel biological drugs will play in the care algorithm.

SUMMARY

AR is driven by an IgE-mediated hypersensitivity to environmental allergens triggering a Th2-mediated response. Current pharmacotherapy for AR is very effective in

Table 2
Studies of other biologics or small molecules targeting type 2 pathways studied in humans

Study	Year	Drug Name and Mechanism	Study Population	End Points	Interesting Points or Problem with Study
Other agents with prospective applications					
Arm JP, Bottoli I, et al[104]	2014	Ligelizumab – Anti-IgE	Atopic patients	Serum IgE levels	
NCT01362244	Ongoing	Mepolizumab - Anti-IL-5	105 CRSwNP patients refractory to conventional therapy	Time to surgery or polyp recurrence after salvage therapy	Will effectively assess duration of action
NCT02772419	Ongoing	Benralizumab – Anti-IL-5 Receptor	Eosinophilic patients with CRS		
NCT02734849	Ongoing	AK001 - Anti-Siglec-8	CRSwNP		Phase 2 RCT
NCT02170337	Ongoing	AMG282 - Anti-IL33/ST2 receptor AMG 157 – Anti-TSLP	41 CRSwNP patients and healthy volunteers Only studied in asthmatic patients and patients with atopic dermatitis	1. Safety 2. Pharmacokinetics	Phase 1 RCT
Small molecule inhibitors of the type 2 pathway					
		SB010 – GATA3 DNAzyme	Only studied in asthmatic patients		
NCT02874144		OC000459 - CRTH2 antagonist Dexpramipexole	AR and asthmatic patients Eosinophil-associated diseases, CRS	Absolute eosinophil levels	

Abbreviations: AR, allergic rhinitis; CRS, chronic rhinosinusitis; CRSwNP, CRS with nasal polyps; CT, computed tomography; Ig, immunoglobulin; IL, interleukin; RCT, randomized clinical trial.

symptom control if guidelines are followed and biologic therapies are subsequently less well studied in AR. CRS is increasingly recognized as a chronic inflammatory process rather than a chronic infection. The type 2 endotype is found in most patients with CRSwNP in Western countries and although CRSsNP is heterogeneous, up to 50% have elevated type 2 inflammation. Novel pharmacotherapies developed to target type 2 inflammation in asthma have been applied to CRSwNP, demonstrating significant promise. However, further investigations are still needed to determine the role, timing, predictive prognostic factors, and long-term effects of these agents.

REFERENCES

1. Fokkens WJ, Lund VJ, Mullol J, et al. EPOS 2012: European position paper on rhinosinusitis and nasal polyps 2012. A summary for otorhinolaryngologists. Rhinology 2012;50(1):1–12.
2. Orlandi RR, Kingdom TT, Hwang PH, et al. International consensus statement on allergy and rhinology: rhinosinusitis. Int Forum Allergy Rhinol 2016;6(Suppl 1): S22–209.
3. Hirsch AG, Stewart WF, Sundaresan AS, et al. Nasal and sinus symptoms and chronic rhinosinusitis in a population-based sample. Allergy 2017;72(2):274–81.
4. Tomassen P, Newson RB, Hoffmans R, et al. Reliability of EP3OS symptom criteria and nasal endoscopy in the assessment of chronic rhinosinusitis–a GA(2) LEN study. Allergy 2011;66(4):556–61.
5. Bent JP 3rd, Kuhn FA. Diagnosis of allergic fungal sinusitis. Otolaryngol Head Neck Surg 1994;111(5):580–8.
6. Ferguson BJ. Eosinophilic mucin rhinosinusitis: a distinct clinicopathological entity. Laryngoscope 2000;110(5 Pt 1):799–813.
7. Lam K, Kern RC, Luong A. Is there a future for biologics in the management of chronic rhinosinusitis? Int Forum Allergy Rhinol 2016;6(9):935–42.
8. Van Zele T, Holtappels G, Gevaert P, et al. Differences in initial immunoprofiles between recurrent and nonrecurrent chronic rhinosinusitis with nasal polyps. Am J Rhinol Allergy 2014;28(3):192–8.
9. Tomassen P, Vandeplas G, Van Zele T, et al. Inflammatory endotypes of chronic rhinosinusitis based on cluster analysis of biomarkers. J Allergy Clin Immunol 2016;137(5):1449–56.e4.
10. Van Zele T, Claeys S, Gevaert P, et al. Differentiation of chronic sinus diseases by measurement of inflammatory mediators. Allergy 2006;61(11):1280–9.
11. Wang X, Zhang N, Bo M, et al. Diversity of TH cytokine profiles in patients with chronic rhinosinusitis: a multicenter study in Europe, Asia, and Oceania. J Allergy Clin Immunol 2016;138(5):1344–53.
12. Bousquet J, Khaltaev N, Cruz AA, et al. Allergic rhinitis and its impact on asthma (ARIA) 2008 update (in collaboration with the World Health Organization, GA(2) LEN and AllerGen). Allergy 2008;63(Suppl 86):8–160.
13. Braido F, Sclifo F, Ferrando M, et al. New therapies for allergic rhinitis. Curr Allergy Asthma Rep 2014;14(4):422.
14. Tan BK, Chandra RK, Pollak J, et al. Incidence and associated premorbid diagnoses of patients with chronic rhinosinusitis. J Allergy Clin Immunol 2013;131(5): 1350–60.
15. Tan BK, Zirkle W, Chandra RK, et al. Atopic profile of patients failing medical therapy for chronic rhinosinusitis. Int Forum Allergy Rhinol 2011;1(2):88–94.

16. Naclerio RM, deTineo ML, Baroody FM. Ragweed allergic rhinitis and the paranasal sinuses. A computed tomographic study. Arch Otolaryngol Head Neck Surg 1997;123(2):193–6.
17. Lidder AK, Detwiller KY, Price CP, et al. Evaluating metrics of responsiveness using patient-reported outcome measures in chronic rhinosinusitis. Int Forum Allergy Rhinol 2017;7(2):128–34.
18. Van Bruaene N, Perez-Novo CA, Basinski TM, et al. T-cell regulation in chronic paranasal sinus disease. J Allergy Clin Immunol 2008;121(6):1435–41, 1441.e1–3.
19. Min JY, Ocampo CJ, Stevens WW, et al. Proton pump inhibitors decrease eotaxin-3/CCL26 expression in patients with chronic rhinosinusitis with nasal polyps: possible role of the nongastric H,K-ATPase. J Allergy Clin Immunol 2017;139(1):130–41.e11.
20. Shaw JL, Fakhri S, Citardi MJ, et al. IL-33-responsive innate lymphoid cells are an important source of IL-13 in chronic rhinosinusitis with nasal polyps. Am J Respir Crit Care Med 2013;188(4):432–9.
21. Nagarkar DR, Poposki JA, Tan BK, et al. Thymic stromal lymphopoietin activity is increased in nasal polyps of patients with chronic rhinosinusitis. J Allergy Clin Immunol 2013;132(3):593–600.e12.
22. Artis D, Spits H. The biology of innate lymphoid cells. Nature 2015;517(7534): 293–301.
23. Saluja R, Khan M, Church MK, et al. The role of IL-33 and mast cells in allergy and inflammation. Clin Transl Allergy 2015;5:33.
24. Kim BS, Wojno ED, Artis D. Innate lymphoid cells and allergic inflammation. Curr Opin Immunol 2013;25(6):738–44.
25. Liu YJ. TSLP in epithelial cell and dendritic cell cross talk. Adv Immunol 2009; 101:1–25.
26. Tan BK, Schleimer RP, Kern RC. Perspectives on the etiology of chronic rhinosinusitis. Curr Opin Otolaryngol Head Neck Surg 2010;18(1):21–6.
27. Mahdavinia M, Carter RG, Ocampo CJ, et al. Basophils are elevated in nasal polyps of patients with chronic rhinosinusitis without aspirin sensitivity. J Allergy Clin Immunol 2014;133(6):1759–63.
28. Kuperman DA, Huang X, Koth LL, et al. Direct effects of interleukin-13 on epithelial cells cause airway hyperreactivity and mucus overproduction in asthma. Nat Med 2002;8(8):885–9.
29. Kato A. Immunopathology of chronic rhinosinusitis. Allergol Int 2015;64(2): 121–30.
30. Stevens WW, Ocampo CJ, Berdnikovs S, et al. Cytokines in chronic rhinosinusitis. Role in eosinophilia and aspirin-exacerbated respiratory disease. Am J Respir Crit Care Med 2015;192(6):682–94.
31. Cao PP, Li HB, Wang BF, et al. Distinct immunopathologic characteristics of various types of chronic rhinosinusitis in adult Chinese. J Allergy Clin Immunol 2009;124(3):478–84, 484.e1–2.
32. Schleimer RP. Immunopathogenesis of chronic rhinosinusitis and nasal polyposis. Annu Rev Pathol 2017;12:331–57.
33. Greiner AN, Hellings PW, Rotiroti G, et al. Allergic rhinitis. Lancet 2011; 378(9809):2112–22.
34. Passalacqua G, Ciprandi G. Novel therapeutic interventions for allergic rhinitis. Expert Opin Investig Drugs 2006;15(12):1615–25.
35. Robinson S, Douglas R, Wormald PJ. The relationship between atopy and chronic rhinosinusitis. Am J Rhinol 2006;20(6):625–8.

36. Harvey R, Hannan SA, Badia L, et al. Nasal saline irrigations for the symptoms of chronic rhinosinusitis. Cochrane Database Syst Rev 2007;(3):CD006394.

37. Snidvongs K, Kalish L, Sacks R, et al. Topical steroid for chronic rhinosinusitis without polyps. Cochrane Database Syst Rev 2011;(8):CD009274.

38. Chong LY, Head K, Hopkins C, et al. Intranasal steroids versus placebo or no intervention for chronic rhinosinusitis. Cochrane Database Syst Rev 2016;(4):CD011996.

39. Kalish L, Snidvongs K, Sivasubramaniam R, et al. Topical steroids for nasal polyps. Cochrane Database Syst Rev 2012;(12):CD006549.

40. Fandino M, Macdonald KI, Lee J, et al. The use of postoperative topical corticosteroids in chronic rhinosinusitis with nasal polyps: a systematic review and meta-analysis. Am J Rhinol Allergy 2013;27(5):e146–57.

41. Penagos M, Compalati E, Tarantini F, et al. Efficacy of mometasone furoate nasal spray in the treatment of allergic rhinitis. Meta-analysis of randomized, double-blind, placebo-controlled, clinical trials. Allergy 2008;63(10):1280–91.

42. Rodrigo GJ, Neffen H. Efficacy of fluticasone furoate nasal spray vs. placebo for the treatment of ocular and nasal symptoms of allergic rhinitis: a systematic review. Clin Exp Allergy 2011;41(2):160–70.

43. Head K, Chong LY, Hopkins C, et al. Short-course oral steroids as an adjunct therapy for chronic rhinosinusitis. Cochrane Database Syst Rev 2016;4: CD011992.

44. Vaidyanathan S, Barnes M, Williamson P, et al. Treatment of chronic rhinosinusitis with nasal polyposis with oral steroids followed by topical steroids: a randomized trial. Ann Intern Med 2011;154(5):293–302.

45. Head K, Chong LY, Hopkins C, et al. Short-course oral steroids alone for chronic rhinosinusitis. Cochrane Database Syst Rev 2016;(4):CD011991.

46. Bachert C, Zhang L, Gevaert P. Current and future treatment options for adult chronic rhinosinusitis: focus on nasal polyposis. J Allergy Clin Immunol 2015; 136(6):1431–40 [quiz: 1441].

47. Ghogomu N, Kern R. Chronic rhinosinusitis: the rationale for current treatments. Expert Rev Clin Immunol 2017;13(3):259–70.

48. Videler WJ, Badia L, Harvey RJ, et al. Lack of efficacy of long-term, low-dose azithromycin in chronic rhinosinusitis: a randomized controlled trial. Allergy 2011;66(11):1457–68.

49. Wallwork B, Coman W, Mackay-Sim A, et al. A double-blind, randomized, placebo-controlled trial of macrolide in the treatment of chronic rhinosinusitis. Laryngoscope 2006;116(2):189–93.

50. Seidman MD, Gurgel RK, Lin SY, et al. Clinical practice guideline: allergic rhinitis. Otolaryngol Head Neck Surg 2015;152(1 Suppl):S1–43.

51. Mostafa BE, Abdel Hay H, Mohammed HE, et al. Role of leukotriene inhibitors in the postoperative management of nasal polyps. ORL J Otorhinolaryngol Relat Spec 2005;67(3):148–53.

52. Vuralkan E, Saka C, Akin I, et al. Comparison of montelukast and mometasone furoate in the prevention of recurrent nasal polyps. Ther Adv Respir Dis 2012; 6(1):5–10.

53. Bousquet PJ, Bachert C, Canonica GW, et al. Uncontrolled allergic rhinitis during treatment and its impact on quality of life: a cluster randomized trial. J Allergy Clin Immunol 2010;126(3):666–8.e1-5.

54. Hellings PW, Fokkens WJ, Akdis C, et al. Uncontrolled allergic rhinitis and chronic rhinosinusitis: where do we stand today? Allergy 2013;68(1):1–7.

55. Baguley C, Brownlow A, Yeung K, et al. The fate of chronic rhinosinusitis sufferers after maximal medical therapy. Int Forum Allergy Rhinol 2014;4(7): 525–32.

56. Lal D, Scianna JM, Stankiewicz JA. Efficacy of targeted medical therapy in chronic rhinosinusitis, and predictors of failure. Am J Rhinol Allergy 2009; 23(4):396–400.

57. Smith TL, Kern R, Palmer JN, et al. Medical therapy vs surgery for chronic rhinosinusitis: a prospective, multi-institutional study with 1-year follow-up. Int Forum Allergy Rhinol 2013;3(1):4–9.

58. Smith KA, Smith TL, Mace JC, et al. Endoscopic sinus surgery compared to continued medical therapy for patients with refractory chronic rhinosinusitis. Int Forum Allergy Rhinol 2014;4(10):823–7.

59. Hopkins C, Rimmer J, Lund VJ. Does time to endoscopic sinus surgery impact outcomes in chronic rhinosinusitis? Prospective findings from the national comparative audit of surgery for nasal polyposis and chronic rhinosinusitis. Rhinology 2015;53(1):10–7.

60. Bachert C, Wagenmann M, Hauser U, et al. IL-5 synthesis is upregulated in human nasal polyp tissue. J Allergy Clin Immunol 1997;99(6 Pt 1):837–42.

61. Gevaert P, Bachert C, Holtappels G, et al. Enhanced soluble interleukin-5 receptor alpha expression in nasal polyposis. Allergy 2003;58(5):371–9.

62. Gevaert P, Lang-Loidolt D, Lackner A, et al. Nasal IL-5 levels determine the response to anti-IL-5 treatment in patients with nasal polyps. J Allergy Clin Immunol 2006;118(5):1133–41.

63. Gevaert P, Van Bruaene N, Cattaert T, et al. Mepolizumab, a humanized anti-IL-5 mAb, as a treatment option for severe nasal polyposis. J Allergy Clin Immunol 2011;128(5):989–95.e1-8.

64. GlaxoSmithKline. Mepolizumab in nasal polyposis. 2009. Available at: https://ClinicalTrials.gov/show/NCT01362244. Accessed March 14, 2017.

65. Bleecker ER, FitzGerald JM, Chanez P, et al. Efficacy and safety of benralizumab for patients with severe asthma uncontrolled with high-dosage inhaled corticosteroids and long-acting beta2-agonists (SIROCCO): a randomised, multicentre, placebo-controlled phase 3 trial. Lancet 2016;388(10056):2115–27.

66. Kolbeck R, Kozhich A, Koike M, et al. MEDI-563, a humanized anti-IL-5 receptor alpha mAb with enhanced antibody-dependent cell-mediated cytotoxicity function. J Allergy Clin Immunol 2010;125(6):1344–53.e2.

67. Kyowa Hakko Kirin Co. L. Study of benralizumab (KHK4563) in patients with eosinophilic chronic rhinosinusitis. 2016. Available at: https://ClinicalTrials.gov/show/NCT02772419. Accessed March 14, 2017.

68. MacGlashan DW Jr, Bochner BS, Adelman DC, et al. Down-regulation of Fc(epsilon)RI expression on human basophils during in vivo treatment of atopic patients with anti-IgE antibody. J Immunol 1997;158(3):1438–45.

69. Adelroth E, Rak S, Haahtela T, et al. Recombinant humanized mAb-E25, an anti-IgE mAb, in birch pollen-induced seasonal allergic rhinitis. J Allergy Clin Immunol 2000;106(2):253–9.

70. Casale TB, Condemi J, LaForce C, et al. Effect of omalizumab on symptoms of seasonal allergic rhinitis: a randomized controlled trial. JAMA 2001;286(23): 2956–67.

71. Chervinsky P, Casale T, Townley R, et al. Omalizumab, an anti-IgE antibody, in the treatment of adults and adolescents with perennial allergic rhinitis. Ann Allergy Asthma Immunol 2003;91(2):160–7.

72. Grundmann SA, Hemfort PB, Luger TA, et al. Anti-IgE (omalizumab): a new therapeutic approach for chronic rhinosinusitis. J Allergy Clin Immunol 2008;121(1): 257–8.
73. Vennera Mdel C, Picado C, Mullol J, et al. Efficacy of omalizumab in the treatment of nasal polyps. Thorax 2011;66(9):824–5.
74. Pinto JM, Mehta N, DiTineo M, et al. A randomized, double-blind, placebo-controlled trial of anti-IgE for chronic rhinosinusitis. Rhinology 2010;48(3): 318–24.
75. Gevaert P, Calus L, Van Zele T, et al. Omalizumab is effective in allergic and nonallergic patients with nasal polyps and asthma. J Allergy Clin Immunol 2013;131(1):110–6.e1.
76. Chandra RK, Clavenna M, Samuelson M, et al. Impact of omalizumab therapy on medication requirements for chronic rhinosinusitis. Int Forum Allergy Rhinol 2016;6(5):472–7.
77. Chipps BE, Figliomeni M, Spector S. Omalizumab: an update on efficacy and safety in moderate-to-severe allergic asthma. Allergy Asthma Proc 2012;33(5): 377–85.
78. Cox L, Platts-Mills TA, Finegold I, et al. American Academy of Allergy, Asthma & Immunology/American College of Allergy, Asthma and Immunology Joint Task Force Report on omalizumab-associated anaphylaxis. J Allergy Clin Immunol 2007;120(6):1373–7.
79. Cox L, Lieberman P, Wallace D, et al. American Academy of Allergy, Asthma & Immunology/American College of Allergy, Asthma & Immunology Omalizumab-Associated Anaphylaxis Joint Task Force follow-up report. J Allergy Clin Immunol 2011;128(1):210–2.
80. Busse W, Buhl R, Fernandez Vidaurre C, et al. Omalizumab and the risk of malignancy: results from a pooled analysis. J Allergy Clin Immunol 2012;129(4): 983–9.e6.
81. Long A, Rahmaoui A, Rothman KJ, et al. Incidence of malignancy in patients with moderate-to-severe asthma treated with or without omalizumab. J Allergy Clin Immunol 2014;134(3):560–7.e4.
82. Li J, Goulding M, Seymour S, et al. EXCELS study results do not rule out potential cancer risk with omalizumab. J Allergy Clin Immunol 2015;135(1):289.
83. Bagnasco D, Ferrando M, Varricchi G, et al. A critical evaluation of anti-IL-13 and anti-IL-4 strategies in severe asthma. Int Arch Allergy Immunol 2016; 170(2):122–31.
84. Bachert C, Mannent L, Naclerio RM, et al. Effect of subcutaneous dupilumab on nasal polyp burden in patients with chronic sinusitis and nasal polyposis: a randomized clinical trial. JAMA 2016;315(5):469–79.
85. Nutku E, Aizawa H, Hudson SA, et al. Ligation of Siglec-8: a selective mechanism for induction of human eosinophil apoptosis. Blood 2003;101(12):5014–20.
86. Kiwamoto T, Kawasaki N, Paulson JC, et al. Siglec-8 as a drugable target to treat eosinophil and mast cell-associated conditions. Pharmacol Ther 2012;135(3): 327–36.
87. Na HJ, Hudson SA, Bochner BS. IL-33 enhances siglec-8 mediated apoptosis of human eosinophils. Cytokines 2012;57(1):169–74.
88. Schleimer RP, Schnaar RL, Bochner BS. Regulation of airway inflammation by Siglec-8 and Siglec-9 sialoglycan ligand expression. Curr Opin Allergy Clin Immunol 2016;16(1):24–30.

89. Allakos I. Study to evaluate multiple doses in patients with nasal polyposis. 2016. Available at: https://ClinicalTrials.gov/show/NCT02734849. Accessed March 17, 2017.

90. Kouzaki H, Matsumoto K, Kato T, et al. Epithelial cell-derived cytokines contribute to the pathophysiology of eosinophilic chronic rhinosinusitis. J Interferon Cytokine Res 2016;36(3):169–79.

91. Reh DD, Wang Y, Ramanathan M Jr, et al. Treatment-recalcitrant chronic rhinosinusitis with polyps is associated with altered epithelial cell expression of interleukin-33. Am J Rhinol Allergy 2010;24(2):105–9.

92. Amgen. A study to evaluate the safety, tolerability, pharmacokinetics, and pharmacodynamics of AMG 282 in healthy subjects and subjects with chronic rhinosinusitis with nasal polyps. 2014. Available at: https://ClinicalTrials.gov/show/NCT02170337. Accessed March 14, 2017.

93. Boita M, Garzaro M, Raimondo L, et al. Eosinophilic inflammation of chronic rhinosinusitis with nasal polyps is related to OX40 ligand expression. Innate Immun 2015;21(2):167–74.

94. Gauvreau GM, O'Byrne PM, Boulet LP, et al. Effects of an anti-TSLP antibody on allergen-induced asthmatic responses. N Engl J Med 2014;370(22):2102–10.

95. Tindemans I, Serafini N, Di Santo JP, et al. GATA-3 function in innate and adaptive immunity. Immunity 2014;41(2):191–206.

96. Sel S, Wegmann M, Dicke T, et al. Effective prevention and therapy of experimental allergic asthma using a GATA-3-specific DNAzyme. J Allergy Clin Immunol 2008;121(4):910–6.e5.

97. Krug N, Hohlfeld JM, Kirsten AM, et al. Allergen-induced asthmatic responses modified by a GATA3-specific DNAzyme. N Engl J Med 2015;372(21):1987–95.

98. Anti-inflammatory agent in sinusitis. Available at: https://ClinicalTrials.gov/show/NCT02874144. Accessed March 14, 2017.

99. Barnes N, Pavord I, Chuchalin A, et al. A randomized, double-blind, placebo-controlled study of the CRTH2 antagonist OC000459 in moderate persistent asthma. Clin Exp Allergy 2012;42(1):38–48.

100. Horak F, Zieglmayer P, Zieglmayer R, et al. The CRTH2 antagonist OC000459 reduces nasal and ocular symptoms in allergic subjects exposed to grass pollen, a randomised, placebo-controlled, double-blind trial. Allergy 2012;67(12):1572–9.

101. Prussin C, Laidlaw TM, Panettieri RA, et al. Dexpramipexole effectively lowers blood and tissue eosinophils in subjects with chronic rhinosinusitis with nasal polyps. J Allergy Clin Immunol.139(2):AB64.

102. Dworetzky SI, Hebrank GT, Archibald DG, et al. The targeted eosinophil-lowering effects of dexpramipexole in clinical studies. Blood Cells Mol Dis 2017;63:62–5.

103. Ference EH, Stubbs V, Lidder AK, et al. Measurement and comparison of health utility assessments in chronic rhinosinusitis. Int Forum Allergy Rhinol 2015;5(10):929–36.

104. Arm JP, Bottoli I, Skerjanec A, et al. Pharmacokinetics, pharmacodynamics and safety of QGE031 (ligelizumab), a novel high-affinity anti-IgE antibody, in atopic subjects. Clin Exp Allergy 2014;44(11):1371–85.

Immunotherapy

Treating with Fewer Allergens?

Cecelia Damask, DO[a,b,]*

KEYWORDS

- Polysensitization • Monosensitization • Allergen sensitization
- Allergy immunotherapy • Multiallergen immunotherapy
- Component resolved diagnostics

KEY POINTS

- Polysensitized individuals can be sensitized to multiple distinct allergens but they can also be sensitized to panallergens shared by many unrelated plants.
- Sensitization to multiple allergens often can be distinguished from sensitization to panallergens by component resolved diagnostics.
- Immunotherapy with a single allergen extract is as effective in polysensitized as in monosensitized patients.
- Some European guidelines recommend that immunotherapy be restricted to the single clinically most bothersome allergen.
- Common US immunotherapy practice is to include in treatment all allergen extracts to which the patient is clinically sensitive.

INTRODUCTION AND BACKGROUND

Allergic rhinitis (AR) and asthma are global health problems for all age groups.[1–6] Allergic rhinitis affects 30 to 60 million individuals annually in the United States, including 10% to 30% of adults and possibly even a higher prevalence in children.[7–9]

Recent surveys requiring a diagnosis of AR confirmed by a physician reported prevalence rates of 14% of US adults and 13% of US children.[10,11] AR is the most common chronic disease in children in the United States today and the fifth most common chronic disease in the United States overall.[12] Previously regarded as a nuisance disorder, AR actually has a significant effect on quality of life and may have considerable consequences if left untreated. Over the years, AR has been trivialized despite its

Disclosures: ALK, Audigy Medical.
[a] Private Practice, Florida Hospital Altamonte Springs, 795 Primera Boulevard Suite 1031, Lake Mary, FL 32746, USA; [b] University of Central Florida College of Medicine, 6850 Lake Nona Boulevard, Orlando, FL 32827, USA
* Lake Mary ENT & Allergy, 795 Primera Boulevard Suite 1031, Lake Mary, FL 32746.
E-mail address: cbaukus@yahoo.com

Otolaryngol Clin N Am 50 (2017) 1153–1165
http://dx.doi.org/10.1016/j.otc.2017.08.012
0030-6665/17/© 2017 Elsevier Inc. All rights reserved.

oto.theclinics.com

prevalence, chronicity, and the burden it imposes on individuals and society.[13,14] AR affects nearly 1 in every 6 Americans and generates $2 to $5 billion in direct health care expenditures annually. Through loss of work and decreased school attendance, AR is responsible for as much as $2 to $4 billion annually in lost productivity.[12]

AR is defined as an immunoglobulin (Ig)E-mediated inflammatory response of the nasal mucous membranes after exposure to inhaled allergens. Symptoms include rhinorrhea (anterior or postnasal drip), nasal congestion, nasal itching, and sneezing. It can be seasonal or perennial, with symptoms being intermittent or persistent.[12] Asthma is a common chronic disorder of the airways that is complex and characterized by variable and recurring symptoms, airflow obstruction, bronchial hyperresponsiveness, and an underlying inflammation. Atopy is the strongest identifiable predisposing factor for developing asthma.[15] Individuals with clinical symptoms of IgE-mediated allergic respiratory disease will have IgE specific to disease-triggering allergens, as demonstrated by skin prick testing (SPT) or serum specific IgE (sIgE) assays.[16]

Polysensitization, or sensitization to more than one allergen, is a common feature of patients with AR.[17] Polysensitization is an immunologic phenomenon that is clinically and epidemiologically relevant and generally more prevalent than monosensitization.[18] The National Health and Nutrition Examination Surveys reported that 38.8% of US participants were polysensitized.[19] It was reported that 12.8% to 25.3% of the participants in the first European Community Respiratory Health Survey were polysensitized.[20] Often most patients consulting otolaryngologists are polysensitized.

Polysensitization has been suggested to be a risk factor for subsequent development of allergic diseases, especially allergic asthma. This has been demonstrated in several longitudinal birth cohort studies, including the Multicenter Allergy Study in Germany, the Manchester Asthma and Allergy Study in the United Kingdom, and the Barn Allergy Milieu Stockholm Epidemiology study in Sweden.[21–24] There is also suggestion that polysensitization may influence the clinical expression of disease with more severe allergic expression being seen in patients with greater number of sensitizations.[25] Asthma is more likely to be associated with AR in polysensitized patients than in monosensitized patients.[16]

However, a polysensitized patient does not necessarily have polyallergy. Polyallergy is defined as a documented, causal relationship between exposure to 2 or more specific, sensitizing allergens and the subsequent occurrence of relevant clinical symptoms of allergy.[16] Approximately 50% to 80% of patients seeking treatment for respiratory allergies are polysensitized, that is, responsive to 2 or more allergens on SPT or in vitro sIgE testing.[26,27] Otolaryngologists must use this information along with the clinical history to determine whether a patient is truly polyallergic, that is, symptomatic due to 2 or more clinically relevant allergens. Allergen immunotherapy treatment strategies for the polysensitized patient vary between the United States and Europe. The predominantly European approach is to treat the single or the 2 most clinically relevant allergen(s), whereas patients in the United States are usually treated for all potential clinically relevant allergens.[28–30]

POLYSENSITIZATION

In the United States, prevalence of allergic sensitization in the general population has been estimated in 3 National Health and Nutrition Examination Surveys (NHANES).[19,31–33] In NHANES II (1976–1980) and III (1988–1994) allergy testing was conducted by SPTs, whereas NHANES 2005 to 2006 measured sIgE levels in serum. The NHANES 2005 to 2006 provides the largest and most recent nationally representative data on IgE-mediated sensitization in the US population.[31] Participants aged

6 years and older were tested for 19 sIgE antibodies, and those ages 1 to 5 years were tested for 9 sIgEs. The NHANES 2005 to 2006 not only tested a greater number of allergens across a wider age range than the prior studies, but also provided quantitative information on extent of allergic sensitization.[31] The threshold for a positive test, which was considered indicative of sensitization, was the level of detection ($\geq$0.35 kUa/L). Among US children 6 years and older, 44.6% tested positive to at least 1 of the 19 allergens and 36.2% of children aged 1 to 5 years old were sensitized to at least 1 of the 9 allergens tested.[31] Although the overall prevalence of sensitization did not differ significantly by census region, there were regional differences for individual allergens and allergen types.[31]

In NHANES III, 10,863 individuals representative of the US population between the ages of 6 and 59 years underwent SPT. One or more positive SPTs were present in 54.3% of those tested individuals. Forty percent of those tested were sensitized to at least 1 outdoor allergen. Of those having a positive SPT result, 71.3% were sensitive to more than 1 allergen with the median number of positive responses being 3.[19] In another study assessing data obtained from the Asthma Clinical Research Network trials, 1338 US patients with mild to moderate asthma received an SPT to 12 allergens or allergen mixes. Ninety-five percent of the subjects had at least 1 positive skin test response. Of these, 14% had positive reactions to 1 or 2 allergens and 81% had positive reactions to 3 or more allergens.[34] SPT was conducted in 11,355 individuals for 9 aeroallergens in the first European Community Respiratory Health Survey. More than 40% of the population had a positive SPT result, with 53% being polysensitized.[20]

Allergy evolves at the clinical level from birth into adulthood. This also has been demonstrated at the level of sensitization. In a cross-sectional, observational study by Melioli and colleagues,[35] the evolution of the IgE repertoire was analyzed. This study documented that atopic infants usually start with monosensitization, that is sensitization to only one class of allergens, but soon tend to become sensitized to other allergens over time. The increasing number of sensitizations seems to characterize the natural history of the allergic patient and may represent a typical evolution of allergy,[35] thus suggesting that polysensitization (ie, sensitization to more than 1 allergen) increases with age. In the French ODISSEE study, the prevalence of polysensitization increased with age, with 54% in children younger than 11 years, 61.7% in adolescents, and 64.8% in adults.[36] In a retrospective study conducted by Purello-D'Ambrosio and colleagues[37] assessing the prevention of new sensitizations in monosensitized subjects treated with specific immunotherapy, after 4 years, 68% of those previously monosensitized had become polysensitized and after 7 years, the prevalence of polysensitization had increased to 77%.

IMMUNOTHERAPY IN POLYSENSITIZED PATIENTS

Some studies suggest there may be a difference between monosensitized and polysensitized patients in their clinical and immunologic responses to allergens. A study of 130 Korean children examined the differences between monosensitized and polysensitized individuals. Allergic indices were examined in 68 monosensitized and 62 polysensitized patients with childhood asthma. Measurements included symptom scores, eosinophil counts, SPTs, serum total and sIgE levels, and interleukin-10 levels. These measurements were used to compare allergic indices between the 2 groups. These children were followed for 18 months after immunotherapy to examine the effectiveness of the treatment. This study found that symptom scores and total IgE levels were significantly higher in the polysensitized group than in the monosensitized group.[38]

Allergen-specific immunotherapy is the only allergen-driven therapy for AR and asthma because it is able to diminish allergic symptoms and reduce the use of medications by inducing clinical and immunologic tolerance to the causal allergen. However, polysensitization may represent a crucial obstacle as far as it concerns the choice of the allergen extract to be used for immunotherapy.[17] A series of real-life, multicenter, observational studies, termed POLISMAIL (Polysensitization Impact on Immunotherapy), was conducted to elucidate the clinical relevance of polysensitizations.[39] These studies also aimed to evaluate the characteristics of polysensitized patients with AR and the behavior of the allergists treating them. The effectiveness and the safety of a 2-year sublingual immunotherapy (SLIT) treatment in such patients were also evaluated. A single allergen extract was used in two-thirds of patients, whereas a mix of 2 allergens was chosen in the remaining one-third. The severity grade of AR and the quality of life (QoL) were significantly improved by immunotherapy in both groups. It is interesting to note that there was no clinical outcome difference between patients treated with mono-allergen SLIT and those treated with multiple-allergen SLIT. This outcome demonstrates that immunotherapy with 1 or 2 allergen extracts can achieve significant improvement in polysensitized patients.

The efficacy of grass-SLIT-tablets in monosensitized and polysensitized patients has been examined. There was no difference in efficacy between those sensitive only to grass and those polysensitized when treated with a 5-grass SLIT tablet[40,41] or a timothy-SLIT tablet.[42]

POLYSENSITIZATION VERSUS POLYALLERGY

It is common practice in the United States to treat polysensitized patients by combining multiple extracts to treat all actual or potential sensitizations.[28–30] In the United States, the average subcutaneous immunotherapy (SCIT) extract preparation contains 8 allergens.[29] An analysis of prescriptions for allergen immunotherapy (AIT) written by US allergists and submitted to an extract laboratory (Greer Laboratories, Lenoir, NC) was performed revealing this mean number of 8 unrelated allergen extracts per prescription.[43] The prevailing approach in Europe is to treat the most clinically significant allergen(s) by using extracts that contain 1, or at most 2, allergens.[28–30] The Allergen Immunotherapy: A Practice Parameter Third Update developed by the Joint Task Force on Practice Parameters emphasizes the allergen immunotherapy extract should contain only clinically relevant allergens in line with the European philosophy.[44] Summary Statement 73 from the AIT practice parameter specifically states that the selection of the components of an allergen immunotherapy extract should be based on a careful history in correlation with positive allergy skin test results or serum sIgE antibodies.[44]

The clinical efficacy of immunotherapy, either SCIT or SLIT, has been supported by numerous clinical trials and meta-analyses.[45] Typically, an immunotherapy trial includes patients sensitized to a single allergen or to other allergens unable to bias the observation. For example, a trial on SCIT or SLIT with a grass pollen extract may include patients sensitized to oak pollen, which has a totally separate season. However, in real life, and especially in adults, most patients are sensitized to multiple allergens, which have exposure overlap. Observational, real-life studies are less methodologically rigorous than randomized controlled trials but are possibly more in line with what is seen in private practice. The POLISMAIL series was performed in a real-life setting and it did confirm that immunotherapy achieved significant improvement in polysensitized patients.[39]

The difference in treatment approaches between the United States and Europe pivots on the debate of whether a polysensitized patient is actually polyallergic. Symptom intensity and duration, unavoidable allergen exposure, and impact on QoL play a role when determining which allergen(s) to treat. In some patients with multiple-allergen sensitizations, the history may not completely elucidate which allergens are clinically significant.[27] Another cited reason for treatment with multiple allergens in the United States is the significant investment of time required for SCIT, due to in-office administration and monitoring after each injection. This fact can make it difficult for US physicians to justify treating only one allergen if there is a possibility that the patient may still remain symptomatic from another allergen after completing immunotherapy for just a single allergen.[27]

PANALLERGENS

Another component in the polysensitization versus polyallergy debate involves allergen cross-reactivity or panallergens. In some polysensitized patients, their responses to multiple allergens on either SPT or in vitro sIgE testing may be explained by allergen cross-reactivity rather than true polyallergy. A polysensitized patient may have developed 1 or more IgE antibodies that react with allergens from several plants. This can occur when IgE antibodies react with structurally similar allergens in botanically closely related species, such as birch and alder or cottonwood and aspen. This also can occur from the development of antibodies to panallergens.

The panallergen concept encompasses families of related proteins (**Table 1**), which are involved in general vital processes and thus, widely distributed throughout nature. Plant panallergens share highly conserved sequence regions, structure, and function. Although originating from unrelated organisms, such functionally related molecules share highly conserved sequence regions and 3-dimensional structures and, hence, can fulfill the requirements for IgE cross-recognition. They are responsible for many IgE cross-reactions even between unrelated pollen and plant food allergen sources.[46] Known panallergens consist of only a few protein families, including profilins, polcalcins, and nonspecific lipid transfer proteins (nsLTPs).

Profilins are important components of the plant cytoskeleton. They represent a family of small (12–15 kDa), highly conserved molecules sharing sequence identities of more than 75% even between members of distantly related organisms.[46] Profilins

Table 1 Homology across families	
Family	**Epitope**
Nonspecific lipid transfer proteins	Ara h 9 Cor a8 Pru p3 Par j 2 Art v 3
Seed storage proteins	2S albumins Ara h 2, 6 and 7 Ber e 1 7S albumins Ara h 1 Gly m 5 11S albumins Ara h 3 Gly m 6 Cor a 9 Gliadins Tri a 19
Pathogenesis-related protein family 10 proteins (PR-10)	Bet v 1 Ara h 8 Gly m 4 Cor a 1 Pru p 1 Agi g 1.01 Mal d 1 Act d 8 Dau c 1
Profilins species	Bet v 2 Pru p 4 Hev b 8 Phl p 12
Calcium-binding proteins	Bet v 4 Phl p 7
Serum albumins	Fel d 2 Can f 3 Bos d 6 Sus PSA Equ c 3
Parvalbumins	Cyp c 1 Gad c 1
Tropomysins	Pen a 1 Der p 10 Ani s 3
Lipocalins	Fel d 1 Fel d 4 Can f 1 Can f 2 Equ c 1 Mus m 1

can be found in all eukaryotic cells and are involved in processes related to cell motility via regulation of microfilament polymerization on binding to actin.[47] Being a component of many essential cellular processes, profilins are ubiquitously spread and can therefore be viewed as panallergens that are responsible for many cross-reactions between inhalant and food allergen sources. Allergenic profilins have been identified in pollen of trees, grasses, and weeds, in plant-derived foods, as well as in latex. IgE cross-reactivity results from the common 3-dimensional profilin fold composed of 2 α-helices and a 5-stranded antiparallel β-sheet, as described for the class of α-β proteins.[47] Due to this conserved structure, profilin-sIgE may cross-react with homologues from virtually every plant source. Profilin sensitization is a risk factor for allergic reactions to multiple pollen and food allergen sources.[48] From 15% to 30% of pollen-allergic subjects become sensitized to profilins encountered in pollens and foods.[49] Polysensitization to different allergen sources is more frequently observed in patients displaying profilin-sIgE antibodies.

The first allergenic profilin was described in birch pollen and was designated Bet v 2.[50] Hazelnut Cor a 2 and Rosaceae profilins (strawberry Fra a 4, apple Mal d 1, cherry Pru av 4, almond Pru du 4, peach Pru p 4, and pear Pyr c 4) are considered to cross-react with grass and birch profilins.[51] Profilins are sensitive to heat denaturation and gastric digestion. Consumption of raw foods by profilin-sensitized patients leads to reactions that are usually restricted to the oral cavity.[52]

Another group of panallergens are called procalcins or polcalcins. Polcalcins are highly cross-reactive calcium-binding allergens that are specifically expressed in pollen tissues. For this reason, sensitization to polcalcins is not associated with an allergy to plant-derived foods.[46] Sensitization to procalcins is found in 5% to 10% of pollen-allergic patients. Sensitization to these panallergens can result in allergic reactions to pollens from a variety of plants.[53]

nsLTPs are composed of a family of proteins that are widely distributed throughout the plant kingdom. These proteins are located in the peel of fruits rather than in the pulp.[54,55] nsLTPs belong to the class of pathogenesis-related (PR) proteins and are thought to play a role in plant defense due to their antifungal and antibacterial activities.[56] PR proteins comprise 14 unrelated protein families.[46]

Cross-reactive carbohydrate determinants (CCDs) are protein-linked carbohydrate structures. CCDs are found as glycoproteins in plants and invertebrate animals (eg, insects such as honey bees and wasps) carrying glycans with carbohydrate determinants that do not exist in mammals. Because these determinants function as foreign epitopes in humans, CCDs are highly immunogenic and can give rise to antibodies such as IgE. CCDs are present in the glycoproteins of virtually all pollens; however, they are probably not clinically significant.[57] It has been reported that more than 20% of allergic patients produce anti-glycan IgE antibodies that bind to glycoproteins in pollen, foods, and insect venoms.[58]

Up to a quarter of patients undergoing in vitro sIgE testing react to these determinants on purified natural allergens; they do not, however, occur on recombinant allergens that are not glycosylated.[59]

Allergen extracts are used for both allergy diagnosis via skin testing and immunotherapy. Currently used allergenic extracts contain mixtures of allergens along with nonallergenic and/or toxic proteins bearing the risk of IgE-mediated side effects and sensitization to new allergens. Moreover, standardization of allergenic extracts still relies on the usage of company-specific units, rendering impossible comparison between commercial allergenic products from different manufacturers. In addition, relevant allergens for a given patient might be underrepresented or even missing in the extract used for diagnosis or therapy.[60] This might be especially true for minor allergens, such as panallergens. However, sensitization to panallergens might worsen the prognosis of allergy due to extensive IgE cross-reactivity toward evolutionary related and unrelated allergen sources or, as in the case of nsLTPs, increase severity of atopic disease. Standardization of allergenic extracts is usually based on the concentration of the main IgE-binding molecule. Therefore, currently available extracts might not be adequate for diagnosing and treating patients reacting to minor allergens. This problem could be solved by molecule-based diagnostics and custom-tailored immunotherapy using a panel of naturally purified or recombinantly produced allergens.

COMPONENT RESOLVED DIAGNOSTICS

Distinguishing between multisensitization and cross-reacting antibodies can be accomplished by in vitro determination of IgE-mediated reactions to panallergens or major allergens. This analysis is termed component resolved diagnostics (CRD) and is performed using purified natural or recombinant allergens that may be tested either with singleplex or multiplex arrays.[59] CRD (molecular allergen diagnostics) is the analysis of individual IgE-reactive biomolecules contained in allergen extracts. CRD can be used to help determine whether clinically irrelevant cross-reactive allergens are the cause of polysensitization.[49,61]

Several studies, all conducted in Europe, have examined the utility of applying CRD to the clinical management of immunotherapy in polysensitized patients. The results of CRD testing in these studies resulted in changes in immunotherapy prescriptions for nearly half the patients.[59] Sensitization in 141 patients with AR/asthma was evaluated by performing a microarray-based panel of 96 allergens. A consensus on the indication for and contents of the immunotherapy prescription based on clinical history and SPT results was obtained on each patient before CRD testing. After CRD testing, agreement with the pretesting recommendations was found in only 46% of patients.[62]

CURRENT GUIDELINES FOR ALLERGEN IMMUNOTHERAPY COMPOSITION

The European Medicines Agency (EMA) has published general guidelines for manufacturers on the preparation and composition of allergen extracts and mixtures of extracts.[63] There is no similar published guidance from the US Food and Drug Administration. The EMA recommends that allergists should mix nonrelated allergens as little as possible and should not mix seasonal and perennial allergens or allergens with proteolytic activity (such as extracts of dust mites, molds, and insects) without justification. Mixing allergens clearly has an impact on pharmaceutical parameters, such as stability and dosing and clinical effects, such as optimal dose and safety.[63] The EMA suggests that the number of allergen extracts in a mixture should be kept to a minimum regardless of the homology/cross-reactivity of the individual extracts.[63]

The Global Allergy and Asthma European Network (GA^2 LEN)/European Academy of Allergology and Clinical Immunology (EAACI) pocket guide[64] offers a comprehensive set of recommendations on the use of immunotherapy in allergic rhinoconjunctivitis and asthma in daily practice. The pocket guide is the result of a consensus reached during several GA^2 LEN/EAACI meetings. The recommendations were compiled following an in-depth review of existing guidelines and publications, including the 1998 EAACI position paper, the 1998 World Health Organization Position Paper on SLIT and the 2001 Allergic Rhinitis and its Impact on Asthma (ARIA), as well as based on the ARIA update 2008, the Sublingual Immunotherapy: World Allergy Organization Position Paper 2009, and the Methodology paper of ARIA. These recommendations state that the number of sensitizations itself is less important than the clinical relevance of each allergen. An individualized approach should be based on the iden-tification of the clinically relevant allergen and should consider the type and severity of symptoms, the longest duration of induced symptoms over the year, the greatest impact on QoL, and how difficult an allergen is to avoid.[64] The GA^2 LEN/EAACI pocket guide does not recommend mixture of allergens in the composition of immunotherapy formulations.[64] The Allergen Immunotherapy: A Practice Parameter Third Update developed by the Joint Task Force on Practice Parameters emphasized that it is important to treat the patients only with relevant allergens.[44]

STUDIES REGARDING MULTIALLERGEN IMMUNOTHERAPY

There have been only a few well-designed, double-blinded, placebo-controlled studies evaluating treatment with multiallergen formulations.[28,65–68] Most meta-analyses published to date have evaluated immunotherapy formulations containing a single allergen or several cross-reactive allergens and have urged caution with re-gard to multiallergen immunotherapy.[16] However, multiallergen immunotherapy is common practice in most allergists' practices in the United States and in 20% to 40% of the prescriptions in Europe.[30]

A review by Nelson[59] identified 13 studies (published between 1965 and 2007) in which 2 or more unrelated allergens were simultaneously administered as subcutane-ous allergen immunotherapy. Seven of these studies used 2 non–cross-reacting aller-gens. Nelson[59] concluded that the clinical outcomes with 2 extracts were superior to those with placebo and equal to those achieved with each as a single-extract treatment.

There are 2 studies in which 2 allergen extracts were administered sublingually via 2 different vials. Both of these studies demonstrated clinical efficacy.[69,70] Fifty-eight patients sensitized to birch and grasses only who had rhinitis and bronchial hyperre-activity in both pollen seasons were enrolled in the study. The patients received SLIT for birch, SLIT for grass, SLIT for birch and grass, or drugs only. Symptom and medi-cation scores, forced expiratory volume in 1 second, bronchial hyperreactivity, and nasal eosinophil counts were evaluated in both pollen seasons at baseline and after 2 and 4 years. Those patients receiving SLIT for grass or birch had a significant clinical improvement and nasal eosinophil reduction versus baseline and versus patients who did not receive SLIT in the target season but also in the unrelated pollen season. The patients receiving SLIT for grass and birch improved as well, and their improvement in clinical symptoms and inflammation was significantly greater than in patients treated with SLIT for the single allergens. In patients sensitized to grass and birch, SLIT with the 2 allergens provided the best clinical results. Nevertheless, SLIT with birch only or grass only also provided a measurable improvement in the grass season and birch season, respectively.[70]

There is only 1 study that examined the use of more than 2 allergens simulta-neously in the same sublingual vial. SLIT was administered for 10 months to 54 pa-tients randomized to 1 of 3 treatment arms: placebo, timothy extract (19 μg Phl p 5 daily) as monotherapy, or the same dose of timothy extract plus 9 additional pollen extracts. Symptom and medication scores were collected and titrated nasal chal-lenges, titrated SPTs, sIgE, IgG4, and cytokine release by timothy-stimulated lymphocyte proliferation were performed. There were no significant differences in medication or symptom scores in either treatment group compared with placebo.[71] However there was a very low grass pollen season in 2008 in that part of the United States due to little rainfall that season and this fact may have contributed to the low symptom scores.[59]

SUMMARY

Immunotherapy with a single allergen is as effective in polysensitized patients as it is in monosensitized patients. Although European guidelines recommend that immunotherapy be limited to the single clinically most troublesome allergen, US physicians tend to include all allergens to which the patient is clinically sensitive in their immunotherapy prescriptions. There are studies that support the effectiveness of SCIT with mixtures of more than 2 unrelated allergen extracts. Most US allergists are convinced of the efficacy of multiple-allergen immunotherapy.

Approximately 50% to 80% of US patients seeking treatment for AR are polysensitized. Otolaryngologists must use these data along with the clinical history to determine whether a patient is truly polyallergic. Some polysensitization represents sensitizations to multiple distinct allergens, but some represent sensitization to panallergens. Sensitization to multiple allergens may be distinguished from sensitization to panallergens by CRD. This may at least in part modify the immunotherapy strategies in the future. Unfortunately, creating a patient's custom-tailored immunotherapy prescription based on recombinant allergens is not available at this time.

REFERENCES

1. Bauchau V, Durham SR. Epidemiological characterization of the intermittent and persistent types of allergic rhinitis. Allergy 2005;60:350–3.
2. Bousquet J, Van CP, Khaltaev N, ARIA Workshop Group, World Health Organization. Allergic rhinitis and its impact on asthma. J Allergy Clin Immunol 2001;108: S147–334.
3. Bousquet J, Khaltaev N, Cruz AA, et al. Allergic rhinitis and its impact on asthma (ARIA) 2008 update (in collaboration with the World Health Organization, GA2LEN and AllerGen). Allergy 2008;63:S8–160.
4. Brozek JL, Bousquet J, Baena-Cagnani CE, et al. Allergic rhinitis and its impact on asthma (ARIA) guidelines: 2010 revision. J Allergy Clin Immunol 2010;126: 466–76.
5. Canonica GW, Bousquet J, Casale T, et al. Sub-lingual immunotherapy: World Allergy Organization position paper 2009. Allergy 2009;64(Suppl 91):1–59.
6. Canonica GW, Cox L, Pawankar R, et al. Sublingual immunotherapy: World Allergy Organization position paper 2013 update. World Allergy Organ J 2014;7:6.
7. Meltzer EO, Bukstein DA. The economic impact of allergic rhinitis and current guidelines for treatment. Ann Allergy Asthma Immunol 2011;106:S12–6.
8. Wallace DV, Dykewicz MS, Bernstein DI, et al. The diagnosis and management of rhinitis: an updated practice parameter. J Allergy Clin Immunol 2008;122:S1–84.
9. Salzano FA, d'Angelo L, Motta S, et al. Allergic rhinoconjunctivitis: diagnostic and clinical assessment. Rhinology 1992;30:265–75.
10. Meltzer EO, Blaiss MS, Naclerio RM, et al. Burden of allergic rhinitis: allergies in America, Latin America, and Asia-Pacific adult surveys. Allergy Asthma Proc 2012;33:S113–41.
11. Meltzer EO. Allergic rhinitis. Burden of illness, quality of life, comorbidities, and control. Immunol Allergy Clin N Am 2016;36(2):235–48.
12. Seidman MD, Gurgel RK, Lin SY, et al. Clinical practice guideline: allergic rhinitis. Otolaryngol Head Neck Surg 2015;152(1 Suppl):S1–43.
13. Price D, Scadding G, Ryan D, et al. The hidden burden of adult allergic rhinitis: UK healthcare resource utilization survey. Clin Transl Allergy 2015;5:39.
14. Bousquet PJ, Demoly P, Devillier P, et al. Impact of allergic rhinitis symptoms on quality of life in primary care. Int Arch Allergy Immunol 2013;160:393–400.

15. National Asthma Education and Prevention Program. Expert panel report 3 (EPR-3): guidelines for the diagnosis and management of asthma-summary report 2007. J Allergy Clin Immunol 2007;120(5 Suppl):S94–138.

16. Demoly P, Passalacqua G, Pfaar O, et al. Management of the polyallergic patient with allergy immunotherapy: a practice-based approach. Allergy Asthma Clin Immunol 2016;12:2.

17. Ciprandi G, Incorvaia C, Puccinelli P, et al. Polysensitization as a challenge for the allergist: the suggestions provided by the polysensitization impact on allergen immunotherapy studies. Expert Opin Biol Ther 2011;11(6):715–22.

18. Ciprandi G, Melioli G, Passalacqua G, et al. Immunotherapy in polysensitized patients: new chances for the allergists? Ann Allergy Asthma Immunol 2012;109(6): 392–4.

19. Arbes SJ Jr, Gergen PJ, Elliott L, et al. Prevalences of positive skin test responses to 10 common allergens in the US population: results from the third National Health and Nutrition Examination Survey. J Allergy Clin Immunol 2005;116: 377–83.

20. Bousquet PJ, Castelli C, Daures JP, et al. Assessment of allergen sensitization in a general population-based survey (European Community Respiratory Health Survey I). Ann Epidemiol 2010;20:797–803.

21. Illi S, von Mutius E, Lau S, et al, Multicentre Allergy Study (MAS) group. Perennial allergen sensitisation early in life and chronic asthma in children: a birth cohort study. Lancet 2006;368(9537):763–70.

22. Custovic A, Sonntag HJ, Buchan IE, et al. Evolution pathways of IgE responses to grass and mite allergens throughout childhood. J Allergy Clin Immunol 2015; 136(6):1645–52.e8.

23. Simpson A, Lazic N, Belgrave DC, et al. Patterns of IgE responses to multiple allergen components and clinical symptoms at age 11 years. J Allergy Clin Immunol 2015;136(5):1224–31.

24. Westman M, Lupinek C, Bousquet J, et al, Mechanisms for the development of allergies consortium. Early childhood IgE reactivity to pathogenesis-related class 10 proteins predicts allergic rhinitis in adolescence. J Allergy Clin Immunol 2015; 135:1199–206.e1-11.

25. Ciprandi G, Alesina R, Ariano R, et al. Characteristics of patients with allergic polysensitization: the POLISMAIL study. Eur Ann Allergy Clin Immunol 2008;40(3): 77–83.

26. Nelson HS, Makatsori M, Calderon MA. Subcutaneous immunotherapy and sublingual immunotherapy: comparative efficacy, current and potential indications, and warnings—United States versus Europe. Immunol Allergy Clin North Am 2016;36:13–24.

27. Pepper AN, Calderón MA, Casale TB. Sublingual immunotherapy for the polyallergic patient. J Allergy Clin Immunol Pract 2017;5(1):41–5.

28. Calderón MA, Cox L, Casale TB, et al. Multiple-allergen and single-allergen immunotherapy strategies in polysensitized patients: looking at the published evidence. J Allergy Clin Immunol 2012;129:929–34.

29. Tabatabaian F, Casale TB. Selection of patients for sublingual immunotherapy (SLIT) versus subcutaneous immunotherapy (SCIT). Allergy Asthma Proc 2015; 36:100–4.

30. Cox L, Jacobsen L. Comparison of allergen immunotherapy practice patterns in the United States and Europe. Ann Allergy Asthma Immunol 2009;103:451–9.

31. Salo PM, Calatroni A, Gergen PJ, et al. Allergy-related outcomes in relation to serum IgE: results from the National Health and Nutrition Examination Survey 2005–2006. J Allergy Clin Immunol 2011;127:1226–35.

32. Gergen PJ, Turkeltaub PC. The association of individual allergen reactivity with respiratory disease in a national sample: data from the second National Health and Nutrition Examination Survey, 1976–80 (NHANES II). J Allergy Clin Immunol 1992;90:579–88.

33. Gergen PJ, Turkeltaub PC, Kovar MG. The prevalence of allergic skin test reactivity to eight common aeroallergens in the U.S. population: results from the second National Health and Nutrition Examination Survey. J Allergy Clin Immunol 1987;80:669–79.

34. Craig TJ, King TS, Lemanske RF Jr, et al. Aeroallergen sensitization correlates with PC(20) and exhaled nitric oxide in subjects with mild-to-moderate asthma. J Allergy Clin Immunol 2008;121(3):671–7.

35. Melioli G, Marcomini L, Agazzi A, et al. The IgE repertoire in children and adolescents resolved at component level: a cross-sectional study. Pediatr Allergy Immunol 2012;23(5):433–40.

36. Didier A, Chartier A, Démonet G. Specific sublingual immunotherapy: for which profiles of patients in practice? Midterm analysis of ODISSEE (observatory of the indication and management of respiratory allergies [rhinitis and/or conjunctivitis and/or allergic asthma] by specific sublingual immunotherapy). Rev Fr Allerg 2010;50:426–33.

37. Purello-D'Ambrosio F, Gangemi S, Merendino RA, et al. Prevention of new sensitizations in monosensitized subjects submitted to specific immunotherapy or not. A retrospective study. Clin Exp Allergy 2001;31:1295–302.

38. Kim KW, Kim EA, Kwon BC, et al. Comparison of allergic indices in monosensitized and polysensitized patients with childhood asthma. J Korean Med Sci 2006;21:1012–6.

39. Ciprandi G, Incorvaia C, Puccinelli P, et al. The POLISMAIL lesson: sublingual immunotherapy may be prescribed also in polysensitized patients. Int J Immunopathol Pharmacol 2010;23:637–40.

40. Malling H-J, Montagut AM, Patriarca G, et al. Efficacy and safety of 5-grass pollen sublingual immunotherapy tablets in patients with different clinical profiles of allergic rhinoconjunctivitis. Clin Exp Allergy 2009;39:387–93.

41. Cox LS, Casale TB, Nayak AS, et al. Clinical efficacy of 300IR 5-gass pollen sublingual tablet in a US study: the importance of allergen-specific serum IgE. J Allergy Clin Immunol 2012;130:1327–34.

42. Nelson H, Blaiss M, Nolte H, et al. Efficacy and safety of the SQ-standardized grass allergy immunotherapy tablet in mono- and polysensitized subjects. Allergy 2013;68:252–5.

43. Esch RE. Specific immunotherapy in the U.S.A.: general concept and recent initiatives. Arb Paul Ehrlich Inst Bundesamt Sera Impfstoffe Frankf A M 2003;94:17–22 [discussion: 23].

44. Cox L, Nelson H, Lockey R, et al. Allergen immunotherapy: a practice parameter third update. J Allergy Clin Immunol 2011;127:S1–55.

45. Compalati E, Penagos M, Tarantini D, et al. Specific immunotherapy for respiratory allergy: state of the art according to current meta-analyses. Ann Allergy Asthma Immunol 2009;102:22–8.

46. Hauser M, Roulias A, Ferreira F, et al. Panallergens and their impact on the allergic patient. Allergy Asthma Clin Immunol 2010;6(1):1.

47. Valenta R, Duchene M, Ebner C, et al. Profilins constitute a novel family of functional plant pan-allergens. J Exp Med 1992;175:377–85.

48. Asero R, Mistrello G, Roncarolo D, et al. Detection of clinical markers of sensitization to profilin in patients allergic to plant-derived foods. J Allergy Clin Immunol 2003;112:427–32.

49. Hamilton RG, Oppenheimer J. Serological IgE analyses in the diagnostic algorithm for allergic disease. J Allergy Clin Immunol Pract 2015;3:833–40.

50. Valenta R, Duchene M, Pettenburger K, et al. Identification of profilin as a novel pollen allergen; IgE autoreactivity in sensitized individuals. Science 1991;253: 557–60.

51. van Ree R, Fernandez-Rivas M, Cuevas M, et al. Pollen-related allergy to peach and apple: an important role for profilin. J Allergy Clin Immunol 1995;95:726–34.

52. Rodriguez-Perez R, Crespo JF, Rodriguez J, et al. Profilin is a relevant melon allergen susceptible to pepsin digestion in patients with oral allergy syndrome. J Allergy Clin Immunol 2003;111:634–9.

53. Kazemi-Shirazi L, Niederberger V, Linhart B, et al. Recombinant marker allergens: diagnostic gatekeepers of the treatment of allergy. Int Arch Allergy Immunol 2001;127:259–68.

54. Fernandez-Rivas M, Cuevas M. Peels of Rosaceae fruits have a higher allergenicity than pulps. Clin Exp Allergy 1999;29:1239–47.

55. Marzban G, Puehringer H, Dey R. Localisation and distribution of the major allergens in apple fruits. Plant Sci 2005;169:387–94.

56. Silverstein KA, Moskal WA Jr, Wu HC, et al. Small cysteine-rich peptides resembling antimicrobial peptides have been under-predicted in plants. Plant J 2007; 51:262–80.

57. Douladiris N, Savvatianos S, Roumpedaki I, et al. A molecular diagnostic algorithm to guide pollen immunotherapy in southern Europe: towards component-resolved management of allergic diseases. Int Arch Allergy Immunol 2013;162: 163–72.

58. Altmann F. The role of protein glycosylation in allergy. Int Arch Allergy Immunol 2007;142:99–115.

59. Nelson HS. Allergen immunotherapy (AIT) for the multiple-pollen sensitive patient. Expert Rev Clin Pharmacol 2016;9(11):1443–51.

60. Egger M, Hauser M, Himly M, et al. Development of recombinant allergens for diagnosis and therapy. Front Biosci 2009;1:77–90.

61. Aalberse RC, Aalberse JA. Molecular allergen-specific IgE assays as a complement to allergen extract-based sensitization assessment. J Allergy Clin Immunol Pract 2015;3:863–9.

62. Sastre J, Landivar ME, Ruiz-Garcia M, et al. How molecular diagnosis can change allergen-specific immunotherapy prescription in a complex pollen area. Allergy 2012;67:709–11.

63. European Medicines Agency. Guideline on allergen products: production and quality issues. London; 2008. EMEA/CHMP/BWP/304831/2007. Available at: www.ema.europa.eu/docs/en_GB/document_library/Scientific_guideline/2009/09/ WC500003333.pdf. Accessed September 17, 2017.

64. Zuberbier T, Bachert C, Bousquet PJ, et al. GA^2 LEN/EAACI pocket guide for allergen-specific immunotherapy for allergic rhinitis and asthma. Allergy 2010; 65(12):1525–30.

65. Nelson HS. Multiallergen immunotherapy for allergic rhinitis and asthma. J Allergy Clin Immunol 2009;123:763–9.

66. Calderon MA, Cox LS. Monoallergen sublingual immunotherapy versus multiallergen subcutaneous immunotherapy for allergic respiratory diseases: a debate during the AAAAI 2013 Annual Meeting in San Antonio, Texas. J Allergy Clin Immunol Pract 2014;2:136–43.
67. Bahceciler NN, Galip N, Cobanoglu N. Multi allergen-specific immunotherapy in polysensitized patients: where are we? Immunotherapy 2013;5:183–90.
68. Passalacqua G. The use of single versus multiple antigens in specific allergen immunotherapy for allergic rhinitis: review of the evidence. Curr Opin Allergy Clin Immunol 2014;14:20–4.
69. Swamy RS, Reshamwala N, Hunter T, et al. Epigenetic modifications and improved regulatory T-cell function in subjects undergoing dual sublingual immunotherapy. J Allergy Clin Immunol 2012;130:215–24.
70. Morogna M, Spadolini I, Massolo A, et al. Effects of sublingual immunotherapy for multiple or single allergens in polysensitized patients. Ann Allergy Asthma Immunol 2007;98:274–80.
71. Amar SM, Harbeck RJ, Sills M, et al. Response to sublingual immunotherapy with grass pollen extract: monotherapy versus combination in a multiallergen extract. J Allergy Clin Immunol 2009;124:150–6.

Advances in Food Allergy

Christine B. Franzese, MD

KEYWORDS

- Food allergy • Biomarkers • Component-resolved testing • Oral challenge
- Peanut allergy • Oral immunotherapy • Sublingual immunotherapy
- Epicutaneous immunotherapy

KEY POINTS

- Improvements in component-resolved testing, biomarkers, and immunoglobulin G 4(IgG4)/IgE ratios may improve practitioner's ability to discriminate between patients who are food sensitive but can tolerate food, and patients who are truly food allergic.
- Studies in oral immunotherapy, sublingual immunotherapy, and epicutaneous immunotherapy show promising results as potential treatment options for food allergy.
- Changes in guidelines regarding the early introduction of foods, particularly peanuts, as well as additional investigations into adjunctive therapies, may help prevent food allergies.

INTRODUCTION

The subject of food allergy continues to gain considerable interest due, in part, to the clinical challenge it presents in diagnosis, treatment, and management. Given its potential to cause life-threatening anaphylactic reactions and its impact on quality of life and health care systems, increasing attention has been directed toward strategies to prevent food allergies, including analysis of populations, genotype, and phenotype risk factors, and timing of the introduction of foods. This article reviews some of the recent advances in the diagnosis, treatment, and prevention of food allergy.

ADVANCES IN DIAGNOSIS

Making the diagnosis of any type of allergy requires the combination of appropriate symptomatic patient history with a positive test for immunoglobulin E (IgE) to relevant antigens. When testing for food-specific IgE either by skin or by serum, the practitioner faces a similar dilemma to testing for other allergens, the dilemma that a positive test indicating sensitization does not necessarily translate to clinically relevant allergy.[1] This reality poses a diagnostic challenge to the provider and sows confusion in the patient who has difficulty reconciling a positive test result to a food he/she consumes

Disclosure: Greer-Speaker's Bureau and Advisory Board; ALK-Advisory Board.
Department of Otolaryngology-Head and Neck Surgery, University of Missouri Medical Center-Columbia, One Hospital Drive, MA314, Columbia, MO 65212, USA
E-mail address: franzesec@health.missouri.edu

Otolaryngol Clin N Am 50 (2017) 1167–1173
http://dx.doi.org/10.1016/j.otc.2017.08.008
0030-6665/17/© 2017 Elsevier Inc. All rights reserved.

without difficulty. In other situations where the test is equivocal or does not meet the threshold to comfortably recommend strict avoidance of the food in question, oral food challenges are employed to determine clinical reactivity, which carry a real risk of potential harm to the patient. When the patient under evaluation is a child, parents also seek to answer the questions of whether the food allergy will be of limited duration or lifelong, whether reactions will be mild or severe, and even whether siblings might develop the same allergy. Improvements in diagnostic testing seek to discriminate between those truly allergic and those merely sensitized without risk of clinical reaction with the goal of reducing the number of oral food challenges needed, as well as predicting duration and severity of food allergy.

Genetic biomarkers may provide 1 method of improving diagnostic accuracy. In a study by Martino and colleagues,[2] 58 food-sensitized patients ages 11 to 15 months and 13 nonallergic controls underwent skin prick testing, specific IgE testing, oral food challenges, and genome-wide DNA methylation profiling of their blood monocytes. Using 96 DNA methylation sites identified from the study group, these biomarkers were used to successfully predict the clinical reactivity and outcomes of oral food challenges with an accuracy of almost 80% (79.2%), surpassing predictive accuracy of both skin prick tests and specific IgE tests.[2] Further development of such biomarkers has the potential to provide clinically useful diagnostic assays to determine which patients are allergic versus sensitized and decrease the need for oral food challenges.

Other possibilities at improving diagnostic accuracy include component-resolved testing and the presence of IgG4 or blocking antibodies. Component-resolved testing is a diagnostic test similar to specific IgE testing, but involves measuring IgE antibodies to specific allergenic molecules that comprise the foods, rather than the crude food extract.[1] In a study of 108 peanut-allergic, 77 peanut-sensitized, and 43 nonallergic/nonsensitized children by Santos and colleagues,[3] assays of specific IgE and IgG4 to peanut and its components were performed. Although peanut-allergic patients had higher levels of specific IgE to peanut and the components Ara h 1, Ara h 2, and Ara h 8, this did not fully explain the clinical differences in reactivity.[3] However, 2 peanut component patterns emerged; all patients sensitized simultaneously to Ara h 1 and to Ara h 2 had peanut allergy, while all patients monosensitized to Ara h 1 were only peanut sensitized.[3]

Peanut IgG4 levels were 1.6-fold higher in peanut-sensitive patients without clinical allergy, but no significant differences between the levels of specific IgG4 to peanut components were seen, except for Ara h 2-specific IgG4, which was higher in peanut-allergic patients. However, the ratio of peanut-specific IgG4 to peanut-specific IgE was 8 times higher in sensitized but tolerant patients, compared with peanut-allergic patients.[3] When the ratio of IgG4 to peanut components was examined, differences between peanut-sensitive but tolerant and peanut-allergic patients became even larger, with the IgG4/IgE ratio to Ara h 1 (18.8-fold, $P = .05$), Ara h 2 (100-fold, $P = .004$), and Ara h 3 (7-fold, $P = .016$).[3] Overall, although the absolute levels of specific IgG and IgE to peanut and its components individually did not fully account for clinical differences in reactivity between peanut-allergic and peanut-sensitive/tolerant patients, the ratios between these 2 antibodies for peanuts and its components did.

Two recent studies by Santos and colleagues[4] have evaluated the usefulness of the basophil activation test (BAT) in discriminating between clinically-allergic and tolerant but sensitized patients, as well as predicting the threshold and severity of response to peanut oral food challenges. In the first study, 43 peanut-allergic, 36 peanut-sensitized but tolerant, and 25 nonallergic children underwent skin prick testing, specific IgE (sIgE) testing to peanut and its components, and BATing. The BAT in peanut-allergic children showed a peanut dose-dependent upregulation of CD63 and CD203c that was not demonstrated in peanut-sensitized but tolerant ($P<.001$) and nonpeanut-sensitized nonallergic children ($P<.001$). Four BAT diagnostic cutoffs showed 97% accuracy, 95% positive predictive value, and 98% negative predictive value, and when combined in a 2-step approach with either skin prick testing or specific IgE testing to Ara 2, reduced the number of food challenges by 97%.[4] In the second study, 124 children underwent skin prick testing, specific IgE testing to peanut and its components, and BAT on the day of an oral food challenge to peanut.[5] The study found that patients with a BAT ratio of CD63 peanut/anti-IgE levels of 1.3 or greater had an increased risk of severe reactions (relative risk [RR], 3.4; 95% confidence interval [CI], 1.8–6.2), and those with a CD-sens value of 84 or greater had an increased risk of reacting to 0.1 g or less of peanut protein (RR, 1.9; 95% CI, 1.3–2.8).[5]

As far as clinic practice, there are no current guidelines or recommendations as to whether component-resolved testing for foods, specific IgG4 levels, or BAT should be ordered. However, these tests can potentially be helpful in guiding clinical decision-making as long as the provider understands that these tests are helpful at making predictions, not definitive determinations at this point in time. Component-resolved testing is not yet available for many foods, while specific IgG4 and BAT may not be widely available anymore. In addition, many insurers consider these tests to be experimental, so if the provider decides to utilize them, the potential costs of each of these tests should be discussed with the patient.

ADVANCES IN TREATMENT

The current mainstay of treatment for food allergy is avoidance and elimination of the allergic food[s] from the patient's diet. Investigation into potential treatments for food allergies has been promising and includes studies into protocols for oral immunotherapy (OIT), sublingual immunotherapy (SLIT), and epicutaneous immunotherapy (EPIT). These protocols, however, are not widely available, and food-allergic patients follow the current standard treatment—avoidance and use of auto-injectable epinephrine with accidental exposures. Other adjuvant therapies, such as Chinese herbal therapy and the use of probiotics, aimed at more general alterations in the immune system, have also received some attention as potential treatments for food allergy, but there are few published sound clinical trials evaluating these.

Oral immunotherapy protocols vary widely in food type used, dosing, and timing of escalation, but essentially all involve mixing the allergic food into a vehicle and consuming it in a sequential, incrementally progressive fashion until a set maintenance dose is reached.[6] In general, oral immunotherapy protocols include an initial dose escalation performed over the course of 1 day, with an minute dose (eg, 0.1 mg of food protein), rapidly increased by doubling doses to a maximum but still subthreshold level of food protein (10–25 mg), in an attempt to identify a dose that be safely given at home.[6] Then a build-up escalation phase is performed with increasing larger doses given every 1 to 2 weeks in the provider's office, with considerable differences in administration between protocols. In between escalation doses in the practitioner's office, the patient continues to take the daily home doses, until a predetermined maintenance dose is reached. There is no set standard for length of escalation (a few months to years) and maintenance dose (300 mg to over 4000 mg of food protein), depending on which food item is used or protocol is being followed.[6]

Although these protocols offer potential treatment options to food-allergic patients, they are limited in that not all patients can tolerate them. Additionally, these protocols are not widely available, are difficult to perform, and appear to induce a transient desensitization of the allergic food rather than the preferred longer-term tolerance. Adverse reactions are also commonly seen in these protocols, with the most common symptoms being oral pruritus and abdominal pain.[6] Some protocols utilize pretreatment with H1 antihistamines, H2 antihistamines, or both, but there is no standard or recommended premedication regimen, and not all protocols use premedication. The protocol withdrawal rates range from 10% to 36%, with the most common adverse event leading to treatment or protocol cessation being abdominal pain and intolerable chronic gastrointestinal symptoms.[6]

SLIT protocols for food allergy are similar in nature to protocols performed for inhalant allergy, in that the allergen is administered in a liquid form, held under the tongue for roughly 2 minutes, and then swallowed. However, sublingual immunotherapy protocols for foods differ in that there tends to be a much more extended period of escalation than for inhalant allergens, and the range of starting dose (usually in micrograms) to maintenance dose (1–10 mg of food protein) is much greater than what is typical with inhalant protocols.[6] Few studies on sublingual immunotherapy for foods have been published, but overall, most sublingual trials seem to have fewer reported adverse events. However, the effects on induced desensitization and elevation of food thresholds to reactivity with food sublingual protocols do not seem to be as great when compared with food oral immunotherapy.[6]

In a 2015 double-blind placebo-controlled trial of 21 patients comparing peanut SLIT and OIT dosing protocols, subjects were escalated to a maintenance dose of 3.7 mg in the SLIT group or 2000 mg in the OIT group.[7] Repeat food challenges were performed after 6 and 12 months of maintenance in both groups. Subjects passing oral food challenges at 12 or 18 months were taken off treatment for 4 weeks and rechallenged. Only 16 of 21 subjects completed the study. Adverse reactions were more common with OIT group, and study discontinuation was generally secondary to gastrointestinal symptoms. All 16 subjects had a greater than tenfold increase in challenge threshold, but threshold elevation was significantly greater in the OIT group compared with that in the SLIT group (141- vs 22-fold).[7] Sustained unresponsiveness was found in only 4 subjects at study completion.[7]

Although studies have demonstrated that skin is a potential route of sensitization in food allergy, it appears it may also be a route of desensitization. Although there are few published studies evaluating EPIT, this technique involves applying an antigen-containing patch to the skin, and there is currently a phase 3 EPIT trial ongoing for peanut and a phase 1/2 EPIT trial for milk underway. The mechanism of action appears to be the activation of skin Langerhans cells with downstream systemic suppression of effector cell responses.[8] There is only 1 fully published EPIT trial that enrolled 18 children with milk allergy in a double-blind placebo-controlled study for 3 months.[9] The oral food challenge threshold after 3 months of treatment showed a trend to desensitization but was not statistically significant.[9]

ADVANCES IN PREVENTION

Although advances have been made in diagnostic techniques and in treatment, a great deal of attention has also been given to preventing the development of food allergies, with much of the attention given to peanut allergy. There is an association of the development of food allergies to atopic dermatitis, and it is thought that cutaneous exposure can serve as a route of sensitization to food allergens, especially if there is disruption of the skin barrier as in the case of atopic dermatitis.[10–12] In a 2015 study comparing peanut protein levels in household dust to skin prick testing, higher levels of peanut protein containing dust increased the odds of peanut sensitization and likely allergy, particularly in households with children with a history of atopic dermatitis.[13]

As it is becoming clearer that sensitization occurs through the cutaneous route, ways to prevent the development of clinical food allergy have turned toward the timing of the introduction of food through the oral route. The LEAP study (Learning Early About Peanut allergy) published in 2015 has since changed guidelines regarding the method of evaluation and timing of introduction of peanut-containing food items in high-, moderate-, and low-risk infants.[14,15] The LEAP study randomly assigned 640 high-risk infants (high risk meaning those with severe eczema, egg allergy, or both) to either consume or avoid peanut-containing food items until 5 years of age. At the end of the study, the prevalence of peanut allergy in those infants with an initial negative skin prick test to peanut was 1.9% in the consumption group and 13.7% in the avoidance group; the prevalence of peanut allergy in those infants with a positive skin test was 10.6% in the consumption group and 35.3% in the avoidance group.[14] This led to the 2017 publication of a guideline addendum from the National Institutes of Allergy and Infectious Diseases,[15] which stated

Infants with severe eczema, egg allergy, or both have introduction of age-appropriate peanut-containing food as early as 4 to 6 months of age. Other solid foods should be introduced before peanut-containing foods to show that the infant is developmentally ready. Evaluation with peanut-specific IgE measurement, SPTs, or both be strongly considered before introduction of peanut to determine if peanut should be introduced and, if so, the preferred method of introduction.

Infants with mild-to-moderate eczema should have introduction of age-appropriate peanut-containing food around 6 months of age, in accordance with family preferences and cultural practices. Other solid foods should be introduced before peanut-containing foods to show that the infant is developmentally ready. These infants may have dietary peanut introduced at home without an in-office evaluation. However, some caregivers and health care providers may desire an in-office supervised feeding, evaluation, or both.

Infants without eczema or any food allergy have age-appropriate peanut-containing foods freely introduced in the diet together with other solid foods and in accordance with family preferences and cultural practices.

In addition to the early introduction of foods, some studies have looked at introducing prebiotics, probiotics, and other nutritional supplements in an attempt to prevent the development of food allergies or conditions associated with food allergy, such as atopic dermatitis. A meta-analysis of 29 randomized trials evaluating the effects of probiotics administered to pregnant women, breast-feeding mothers, and/or infants demonstrated that probiotics reduced the risk of eczema when taken by women during the third trimester, when taken by breast-feeding mothers, and when given to infants, but there was no demonstrable effect on other allergic conditions and the certainty in the evidence grading was low.[16] Another randomized trial of 414 infants in a prebiotic formula group, 416 infants in a regular formula group, and 300 breast-fed infants demonstrated significantly decreased development of atopic dermatitis in the prebiotic formula group compared with the regular formula group (5.7% versus 9.7%) at 12 months of age.[17] However, this effect has not been demonstrated to persist beyond 1 year of age.

Overall, there have been a significant number of studies looking at methods to improve diagnosis, treatment, and prevention of food allergies. Undoubtedly in the next few years, not only will additional clinical diagnostic tests become more widely available to aid in the differentiation between food-allergic and sensitive but tolerant patients, but methods of desensitization, such as epicutaneous immunotherapy, will become more viable alternatives to avoidance. As the general understanding of food allergy improves, strategies for the prevention of food allergy will become more successful.

REFERENCES

1. Muraro A, Werfel T, Hoffmann-Sommergruber K, et al, EAACI Food Allergy and Anaphylaxis Guidelines Group. EAACI Food Allergy and Anaphylaxis Guidelines. Diagnosis and management of food allergy. Allergy 2014;69:1008–25.
2. Martino D, Dang T, Sexton-Oates A, et al. Blood DNA methylation biomarkers predict clinical reactivity in food-sensitized infants. J Allergy Clin Immunol 2015;135:1319–28.
3. Santos AF, James LK, Bahnson HT, et al. IgG4 inhibits peanut-induced basophil and mast cell activation in peanut-tolerant children sensitized to peanut major allergens. J Allergy Clin Immunol 2015;135:1249–56.
4. Santos AF, Douiri A, Becares N, et al. Basophil activation test discriminates between allergy and tolerance in peanut-sensitized children. J Allergy Clin Immunol 2014;134:645–52.
5. Santos AF, Du Toit G, Douiri A, et al. Distinct parameters of the basophil activation test reflect the severity and threshold of allergic reactions to peanut. J Allergy Clin Immunol 2015;135:179–86.
6. Wood RA. Food allergen immunotherapy: current status and prospects for the future. J Allergy Clin Immunol 2016;137:973–82.
7. Narisety SD, Frischmeyer-Guerrerio PA, Keet CA, et al. A randomized, double-blind, placebo-controlled pilot study of sublingual versus oral immunotherapy for the treatment of peanut allergy. J Allergy Clin Immunol 2015;135:1275–82.e1-6.
8. Mondoulet L, Dioszeghy V, Thebault C, et al. Epicutaneous immunotherapy for food allergy as a novel pathway for oral tolerance induction. Immunotherapy 2015;7:1293–305.
9. Dupont N, Kalach P, Soulaines S, et al. Cow's milk epicutaneous immunotherapy in children: a pilot trial of safety, acceptability, and impact on allergic reactivity. J Allergy Clin Immunol 2010;125:1165–7.
10. Lack G, Fox D, Northstone K, et al, Avon Longitudinal Study of Parents and Children Study Team. Factors associated with the development of peanut allergy in childhood. N Engl J Med 2003;348:977–85.
11. Du Toit G, Tsakok T, Lack S, et al. Prevention of food allergy. J Allergy Clin Immunol 2016;137:998–1010.
12. Tsakok T, Marrs T, Mohsin M, et al. Does atopic dermatitis cause food allergy? A systematic review. J Allergy Clin Immunol 2016;137:1071–8.
13. Brough HA, Liu AH, Sicherer S, et al. Atopic dermatitis increases the effect of exposure to peanut antigen in dust on peanut sensitization and likely peanut allergy. J Allergy Clin Immunol 2015;135:164–70.
14. Du Toit G, Roberts G, Sayre PH, et al. Randomized trial of peanut consumption in infants at risk for peanut allergy. N Engl J Med 2015;372:803–13.
15. Togias A, Cooper SF, Acebal ML, et al. Addendum guidelines for the prevention of peanut allergy in the United States: report of the National Institute of Allergy

and Infectious Diseases-sponsored expert panel. J Allergy Clin Immunol 2017; 139:29–44.

16. Cuello-Garcia CA, Brozek JL, Fiocchi A, et al. Probiotics for the prevention of allergy: a systematic review and meta-analysis of randomized controlled trials. J Allergy Clin Immunol 2015;136:952–61.

17. Gruber C, van Stuijvenberg M, Mosca F, et al. Reduced occurrence of early atopic dermatitis because of immunoactive prebiotics among low-atopy-risk infants. J Allergy Clin Immunol 2010;126:791–7.

Management of Anaphylaxis

Stella E. Lee, MD

KEYWORDS

- Anaphylaxis • Epinephrine • Subcutaneous immunotherapy • Allergic rhinitis
- Asthma

KEY POINTS

- Cutaneous manifestations including urticaria, angioedema, and flushing are the most common physical examination findings in anaphylaxis.
- Intramuscular epinephrine should be administered in any patient suspected of having an anaphylactic episode with 0.2 to 0.5 mL at a concentration of 1:1000 for adults and 0.01 mg/kg in pediatric patients.
- Serum tryptase is currently the most helpful laboratory test to evaluate for anaphylaxis, although other tests are investigated that may increase the sensitivity of testing.
- Patients receiving subcutaneous immunotherapy should be observed for at least 30 minutes after injection. Screening for asthma and dose reduction during pollen season may decrease the risk of anaphylaxis.

INTRODUCTION
Definition and Epidemiology

Although first described in 1901, a meaningful and accurate definition of anaphylaxis is still being refined. Anaphylaxis is defined as a severe systemic reaction that is potentially fatal and caused by exposure to an allergy-causing substance.[1] The lifetime risk of anaphylaxis in the US population is approximately 1.6% and the frequency of hospital admissions are reportedly increasing, likely owing to the increase seen in food allergy, although mortality has slightly decreased.[2,3]

The causes of anaphylaxis are complex and diverse, including foods, medications, insect stings, and systemic mast cell degranulating disorders. Food triggers are the most common cause of anaphylaxis, followed by medications, and hospital admissions for food-related anaphylaxis in children more than doubled from 2000 to 2009.[4] The most common foods that cause anaphylaxis are peanuts, tree nuts, shellfish, fish, egg, and cow's milk.[5] Risk factors for fatal food-related anaphylaxis include

Department of Otolaryngology–Head and Neck Surgery, University of Pittsburgh Medical Center, Mercy Hospital, 1400 Locust Street, Building B, Suite 11500, Pittsburgh, PA 15219, USA
E-mail address: Lees6@upmc.edu

Otolaryngol Clin N Am 50 (2017) 1175–1184
http://dx.doi.org/10.1016/j.otc.2017.08.013
0030-6665/17/© 2017 Elsevier Inc. All rights reserved.

oto.theclinics.com

adolescent age, history of allergy to peanuts or tree nuts, asthma, and patients without obvious cutaneous symptoms.

The 2 most common medications causing anaphylaxis are antibiotics (beta-lactam) and nonsteroidal antiinflammatory drugs.[2,5] Testing for medication-induced anaphylaxis remains lacking and history continues to be important in determining the etiology. The most common etiology for anaphylaxis in the allergy office is the administration of subcutaneous immunotherapy (SCIT), which warrants appropriate training and continued education of staff, as well as preparedness to treat this potentially fatal reaction.

DIAGNOSIS OF ANAPHYLAXIS
Signs and Symptoms of Anaphylaxis

Cutaneous manifestations are the most common, with urticaria and angioedema occurring in up to 90% of patients and flushing of the skin in more than one-half of patients.[6] It is uncommon for patients to have pruritus without urticaria. Respiratory symptoms include dyspnea or wheezing is seen in approximately 50% of patients and upper airway angioedema in more than one-half of all patients. Gastrointestinal symptoms such as nausea, vomiting, diarrhea, and discomfort can also occur, and have been reported in approximately one-third of patients. Hypotension and shock occur in severe episodes.

Elements of the history that are important to obtain in patients suspected of experiencing anaphylaxis include foods and medications ingested within 6 hours of the episode, activity during the episode, duration, time of day, location, stings or bites, heat or cold exposure, associated symptoms, recurrence of symptoms, and treatment provided.[5]

Differential Diagnosis of Anaphylaxis

Several other conditions can present with symptoms similar to anaphylaxis, including vasovagal reactions and disorders that cause flushing of the skin, angioedema, and/ or vocal cord dysfunction. Vasovagal reactions are quite common and should be differentiated from anaphylaxis. Pallor, diaphoresis, bradycardia, hypotension, and a lack of cutaneous manifestations such as urticaria, pruritus, angioedema, and flushing characterize vasovagal reactions. Bradycardia can also occur during anaphylaxis, but tachycardia is often a precursor to bradycardia in an anaphylactic episode.[5]

Flushing of the skin can be caused by medications such as niacin, angiotensin-converting enzyme inhibitors, vancomycin, and ingestants such as alcohol, monosodium glutamate, and scombroid fish. Scombroidosis occurs after consuming spoiled fish containing increased levels of histamine. In these cases the tryptase levels would be normal.[7] Other syndromes such as mastocytosis, carcinoid, vasointestinal polypeptide tumors, and medullary carcinoma of the thyroid can cause flushing of the skin that may be confused with anaphylaxis.

Tests that can help to establish a diagnosis of anaphylaxis during or in the immediate subsequent period include serum tryptase, histamine, 24-hour urinary histamine metabolites, and urinary prostaglandin D2. Typically, serum tryptase is considered the most helpful test to establish a diagnosis of anaphylaxis, although studies have shown that plasma histamine levels, cysteinyl leukotrienes, and prostaglandins may be more sensitive and remain under further investigation.[8] Tryptase peaks up to an hour and a half after the initial onset of anaphylaxis and can remain elevated several hours afterward.

Tests to identify the cause of anaphylaxis include skin and in vitro testing to identify specific immunoglobulin E to foods and medications. Using fresh food for skin prick testing can be more sensitive than commercially developed extracts. Because foods are the most common cause of anaphylaxis, it is recommended that anyone experiencing an anaphylaxis episode be tested for hypersensitivity to the most common food triggers. If there is delayed anaphylaxis occurring several hours after a meal, especially in the setting of a possible tick bite and ingestion of meat, testing should be considered for immunoglobulin E to galactose-alpha-1,3-galactose, which is present in the tissue of nonhuman mammals. A commercially available benzylpenicilloyl polylysine skin test can be useful to evaluate for penicillin allergy in adults and in children with a negative predictive value of 95% to 99%, although history can obviate the need for testing in low-risk patients.[9,10]

Mastocytosis and mast cell–activating disorders can also be the cause of anaphylactic episodes. These patients often have elevated baseline serum tryptase, histamine, 24-hour urine histamine metabolites, and/or prostaglandin D2. Although a tryptase level of 20 ng/mL has been conventionally used as a cutoff level for diagnosis, lower levels can be present. A blood test screening for the 816V mutation can be helpful for the diagnosis of mastocytosis, but bone marrow biopsy currently is the definitive method to establish the diagnosis.[11,12] Other methods of testing under investigation include component-resolved diagnosis and basophil activation tests, which in the future may be able to provide a more accurate diagnosis.

TREATMENT OF ANAPHYLAXIS
Early Epinephrine Administration

Prompt recognition of anaphylaxis symptoms with appropriate treatment is critical to minimizing mortality. The most important first-line therapy for anaphylaxis is intramuscular injection of epinephrine. Epinephrine should be administered in the midlateral thigh (vastus lateralis muscle), the inciting allergen should be removed if possible, and the patient should be assessed for airway, breathing, circulation, and mental status.[2,5,13,14] In the office setting, appropriate assistance should be sought immediately from appropriate staff and emergency medical personnel.

The dose of epinephrine is 0.2 to 0.5 mL at a concentration of 1:1000 for adults. The pediatric dose is 0.01 mg/kg with a maximum dose of 0.3 mg. Patients with severe symptoms should be provided a higher dose and repeat dosing can be administered every 5 to 15 minutes in conjunction with establishing intravenous access and transfer to a higher level of intensive care if required. In more than one-third of patients, a repeat dose was required to adequately treat an anaphylactic episode.[15]

Epinephrine is the first choice of medical therapy in anaphylaxis owing to its alpha-1 agonist effects that can help to prevent and treat airway edema, hypotension, and shock, as well as its beta-1 agonist effects on cardiac function and beta-2 agonist effects leading to bronchodilation.[16–19] Early administration of epinephrine, defined as before arriving in the emergency department, has been associated with decreased hospitalization (17% vs 43%; $P<.001$) in a study of 384 emergency visits.[20] Delayed epinephrine administration has been associated with fatal anaphylaxis with only 23% of patients receiving the medication before cardiac arrest and, in another study, epinephrine was used correctly in only 47% of fatalities (9 of 19 patients).[21,22] As of this writing, there is no absolute contraindication to the use of epinephrine in a patient suspected of having anaphylaxis.

Other immediate measures to be taken include placing the patient in a recumbent position. Pregnant women should be placed in the left lateral position. Vital signs including pulse oximetry should be used if available and oxygen provided if needed. Oxygen is considered the second important therapeutic intervention after epinephrine and critical for all patients experiencing anaphylaxis, especially in the patient experiencing respiratory or cardiovascular effects. A facemask can be used to deliver 100% oxygen at a rate of 6 to 10 L/min to keep oxygen saturation at greater than 93%.[5,19] Intravenous access should be established for fluid and medication administration if required. Fluid replacement with 1 to 2 L of 0.9% normal saline within 5 minutes for adults and up to 30 mL/kg in the first hour for children may be necessary for hypotension.

Additional measures include albuterol via nebulizer for lower airway obstruction, such as symptoms of wheezing, coughing, and shortness of breath. The adult dose is 2.5 to 5.0 mg/3 mL in saline and 2.5 mg/3 mL in children. Glucagon is indicated for patients who are on beta-adrenergic blockers and are not responsive to epinephrine. Glucagon 1 to 5 mg can be given intravenously over 5 minutes. The mechanism of action is by direct activation of adenyl cyclase, bypassing the beta-adrenergic receptor.

Refractory anaphylaxis has been observed in patients who are on beta-adrenergic blocker therapy, including ophthalmic medications. The symptoms described are paradoxic bradycardia, hypotension secondary to decreased cardiac contractility, and persistent bronchospasm.[23,24] Unfortunately, patients who are on selective beta-1 antagonists do not have a lower risk of anaphylaxis because both beta-1 and beta-2 antagonists can inhibit the receptor. Patients who are on beta-blocker therapy may also have symptoms more resistant to epinephrine therapy and unopposed alpha-adrenergic stimulation, leading to significant hypertension.

The intravenous administration of epinephrine can be provided for patients not responding to intramuscular epinephrine, by adding 1 mg (1 mL of 1:000) epinephrine to 1 L of 0.9% normal saline and providing 2 μg/min (2 mL/min) to be titrated up to 10 μg/min (10 mL/min) if required.[2,5] Intraosseous access can be used if intravenous access is not possible for administration of intravenous fluids and epinephrine. Patients who develop laryngeal edema may require endotracheal intubation or emergent cricothyroidotomy in severe cases when ventilation by bag–mask is ineffective. Vasopressors such as dopamine are indicated in addition to epinephrine if the patient is unresponsive to the treatments discussed. These interventions would be performed in a monitored setting if possible.

Second-line therapies include H1 antihistamines and corticosteroids, although efficacy in the emergent setting has not been established for these medications. Guidelines concur that these medications should not be used as a first-line or sole therapy.[2,5,16,17] Although H1 antihistamines are effective for allergic symptoms such as rhinitis, pruritus, and urticaria, they are not effective in treating airway obstruction or cardiovascular compromise. The use of H2 antihistamines is not supported by the evidence in the literature and may increase hypotension. Both medical professionals and patients alike may delay the administration of epinephrine owing to the misconception that the antihistamine may help to treat anaphylaxis, resulting in increased severity of symptoms and death. The evidence for corticosteroids in treating the biphasic or prolonged episodes of anaphylaxis has been extrapolated from asthma data, and these medications should not be used as initial therapy for anaphylaxis.[16,19] Corticosteroids have an onset of action of between 4 and 6 hours, and dosing is typically 1 to 2 mg/kg per dose of methylprednisolone or equivalent.

Monitoring and Education after Anaphylaxis

The decision for monitoring should be based on symptom severity and risk factors. Hospital admission should be considered in patients who have upper or lower airway edema, prolonged symptoms, when an allergen has been ingested, risk factors for severe anaphylaxis such as asthma, and/or when more than 1 dose of epinephrine was required to treat the patient.[5,17,18] A study of 541 patients diagnosed with anaphylaxis showed that 4% (21 patients) developed biphasic reactions with a median time of 7 hours from the initial onset of symptoms to the onset of the biphasic reaction.[25] In this study, increased risk was associated with history of prior anaphylaxis, an unknown cause of anaphylaxis, or symptoms of diarrhea or wheezing. Biphasic reactions in the literature have been reported to range from 0.4% to 23.0%.[25,26] Monitoring should be individualized to the patient's risk factors, reliability, and access to care.

Upon discharge from medical care patients should be prescribed an epinephrine autoinjector and educated regarding proper use. At least 2 doses should be provided; about one-third of patients will require a second dose of epinephrine to treat anaphylaxis.[15,27] Commercially available autoinjectors are provided in 0.15-mg and 0.30-mg formulations. An identification bracelet or equivalent should be worn and an anaphylaxis action plan should be provided to the patient. There are examples available on the websites of the American Academy of Allergy, Asthma, and Immunology and the American Academy of Pediatrics. Referral should be provided to an allergist or an immunologist for further management.

Prevention of Anaphylaxis

It is difficult to predict the severity of future anaphylaxis episodes based on prior events, and diagnostic testing is inadequate to predict anaphylaxis severity. Patients who are diagnosed with hypersensitivity to a specific trigger such as a food, medication, or insect sting should be counseled on avoidance measures. Education regarding reading food labels carefully including possible hidden sources of the food trigger can be helpful. Currently, desensitization to foods is still under investigation and avoidance is recommended. Cross-reactivity between allergens in foods as well as in medications can trigger reactions, and appropriate education and counseling should be provided regarding avoidance measures.

If a patient will be exposed to a known trigger for systemic reaction, such as radiocontrast material or to prevent recurrent episodes of idiopathic anaphylaxis, it is reasonable to use pharmacologic prophylaxis such as treatment with antihistamines and corticosteroids. Pretreatment for patients sensitive to radiocontrast material is 50 mg of prednisone orally before exposure (at 13 hours, 7 hours, and at 1 hour) and 50 mg of diphenhydramine 1 hour before administration.[28]

Patients who have anaphylaxis to insect stings may be candidates for desensitization via immunotherapy. Skin testing to venom should be performed in patients who have experienced anaphylaxis from "flying hymenoptera" and to whole-body extract for bites from a fire ant. Baseline tryptase levels should be performed in all patients who have had anaphylaxis from a hymenoptera sting to rule out systemic mastocytosis. Venom immunotherapy is 80% to 98% effective and, therefore, should be considered in patients with prior systemic reactions.[5,18]

Because epinephrine is the single most important medication for the early treatment of anaphylaxis and prevention of possible complications, appropriate counseling on carrying an epinephrine autoinjector at all times and its correct use should be provided.

Anaphylaxis to Subcutaneous Immunotherapy

Allergen immunotherapy is the only disease-modifying treatment of allergic disease and is efficacious for symptom relief, decreased need for medications, prevention of new sensitizations, and the prevention of asthma.[29–31] The most serious side effect of SCIT, however, is anaphylaxis, with symptoms ranging from mild pruritus and urticaria to death. The World Allergy Organization has developed a grading system ranging from 1 to 5 to systematically characterize reactions from SCIT (**Table 1**).[32] Fatalities from SCIT-related anaphylaxis are rare, with estimates of approximately 3.4 deaths per year or 1 in every 2.5 million injections.[33] A recent surveillance study evaluating data from 2008 to 2013 on 28.9 million injection visits for 344,480 patients reported a total of 4 fatalities from SCIT and no fatalities reported for sublingual immunotherapy.[34] Systemic reactions occurred in 1.9% of patients on SCIT (grade 3, 0.08%; grade 4, 0.02%) and 1.4% of patients on off-label sublingual immunotherapy (grade 3, 0.03%; grade 4, 0%). The study also confirmed that screening for asthma and dose reduction during peak pollen seasons may help to decrease the risk of systemic reactions. One of the fatalities described occurred under the care of an otolaryngologist during the surveillance period 2012 to 2013 in which a patient left the office without complying with the recommended observation period. The patient collapsed outside the office and died shortly after the anaphylaxis episode. Epinephrine was not available and, therefore, not administered for this patient. It was also reported that the patient had asthma, but it is unknown regarding the level of the patient's asthma control or severity. This fatality does highlight the importance of observing patients after the injection as well as the importance of expedient administration of epinephrine by trained personnel when anaphylaxis occurs. Most severe anaphylactic episodes occur within 30 minutes of an injection. It is recommended that allergy injections be provided in a supervised clinic setting with personnel trained in the recognition and treatment of anaphylaxis.[5,19,30,34] The office should be prepared with epinephrine, oxygen, and methods to maintain an airway and to establish intravenous access for fluids and medications. It is not recommended that allergy injections be administered at home secondary to the risks of anaphylaxis, with the rare exception when the benefits may outweigh the risks, such as in life-threatening hypersensitivity reactions to stinging insects.[30] The assessment of asthma control should be done before each injection because most fatal reactions occur in patients who have uncontrolled asthma.[5,30,33] Anaphylaxis related to angiotensin-converting enzyme inhibitors and SCIT have been reported in a few case reports with hymenoptera venom immunotherapy. Severe hypotension occurred within minutes of the injection, but fortunately all patients were successfully resuscitated and also could resume immunotherapy without a reaction when the angiotensin-converting enzyme inhibitor was held

Table 1	
World Allergy Organization subcutaneous immunotherapy systemic reaction grading system	
Grade	**Description of Criteria**
1	Pruritus, urticaria, angioedema (not upper airway), rhinitis, throat clearing, cough, nausea, headache
2	Asthma responding to an inhaled bronchodilator or gastrointestinal symptoms or uterine cramps
3	Asthma not responding to an inhaled bronchodilator or laryngeal, uvular, or tongue angioedema
4	Respiratory failure with or without loss of consciousness or hypotension with or without loss of consciousness
5	Death

Adapted from Cox L, Larenas-Linnemann D, Lockey RF, et al. Speaking the same language: The World Allergy Organization subcutaneous immunotherapy systemic reaction grading system. J Allergy Clin Immunol 2010;125(3):571; with permission.

Table 2		
First-line anaphylaxis medications and supplies		
Basic Supplies	**Airway and IV Resuscitation Equipment**	**Medications**
Stethoscope	Bag–valve–mask	Epinephrine 1:1,000, 3 doses
Blood pressure cuff	Face masks	or 1 multidose vial
Pulse oximeter	Oropharyngeal airways	O_2 E-cylinder >1100 psi
IV catheters (14-, 16-, 18-,	Nasal pharyngeal airways	Albuterol inhalational
20-, and 22-gauge)	O_2 nasal cannula and tubing	solution 0.5%
IV butterfly needles (19-, 21-,	IV administration set and	Glucagon 1 mg/mL (2 vials)
and 23-gauge)	connection tubing	
Syringes (1, 10, and 20 mL)	Nebulizer with face mask,	
Needles (1–2 inches, 18-, 21-,	tubing	
and 23-gauge)		
Latex-free gloves		

Abbreviation: IV, intravenous.
Adapted from Lieberman P, Nicklas RA, Randolph C, et al. Anaphylaxis–a practice parameter update 2015. Ann Allergy Asthma Immunol 2015;115(5):362; with permission.

for at least 24 hours before injection.[35,36] Whether all patients on SCIT should be prescribed and required to carry an epinephrine autoinjector is controversial and remains at the discretion of the treating physician.

OTOLARYNGIC ALLERGY OFFICE PREPARATION FOR ANAPHYLAXIS

Education of office staff regarding recognition and expedient treatment of anaphylaxis is important to prevent progression of symptoms and mortality. Prompt recognition of a systemic reaction and early use of epinephrine can be life saving. Quality improvement programs that stress continued education, development of a standardized protocol, safety checks, and mock anaphylaxis drills can help to decrease the risk of anaphylaxis related to SCIT administration.[37–39] In addition, informed consent and a written contract with the patient regarding the risks of allergy testing, SCIT, and the required postinjection wait time can be helpful to educate the patient regarding the risks of treatment and establish standardized care. Important first-line medications and supplies to treat anaphylaxis adapted from recent practice parameters are listed in **Table 2**. Development of an office action plan for the management of anaphylaxis is also critical to appropriately treat the patient in an emergent setting.

SUMMARY

Anaphylaxis can present in many forms with varied etiologies. Prompt diagnosis and early treatment with epinephrine is critical to minimizing mortality. There is no absolute contraindication to providing epinephrine for a patient suspected of experiencing anaphylaxis. Once a diagnosis of anaphylaxis is established, patients should be appropriately counseled on preventive strategies; advances in diagnosis and treatment continue to evolve for the management of anaphylaxis, especially in the areas of food allergy, desensitization, and understanding mast cell disorders. In the allergy office, proactive measures to improve safety can decrease anaphylaxis and improve quality of care. Recent surveillance data highlight the importance of postinjection wait times and the potential to decrease risk of anaphylaxis by screening for asthma control, as well as dose reduction during peak pollen season.

REFERENCES

1. Sampson HA, Munoz-Furlong A, Campbell RL, et al. Second symposium on the definition and management of anaphylaxis: summary report–second National Institute of Allergy and Infectious Disease/Food Allergy and Anaphylaxis Network symposium. J Allergy Clin Immunol 2006;117(2):391–7.
2. Simons FE, Ebisawa M, Sanchez-Borges M, et al. 2015 update of the evidence base: World Allergy Organization anaphylaxis guidelines. World Allergy Organ J 2015;8(1):32.
3. Wood RA, Camargo CA Jr, Lieberman P, et al. Anaphylaxis in America: the prevalence and characteristics of anaphylaxis in the United States. J Allergy Clin Immunol 2014;133(2):461–7.
4. Rudders SA, Arias SA, Camargo CA Jr. Trends in hospitalizations for food-induced anaphylaxis in US children, 2000-2009. J Allergy Clin Immunol 2014; 134(4):960–2.e3.
5. Lieberman P, Nicklas RA, Randolph C, et al. Anaphylaxis–a practice parameter update 2015. Ann Allergy Asthma Immunol 2015;115(5):341–84.
6. Lieberman P, Nicklas RA, Oppenheimer J, et al. The diagnosis and management of anaphylaxis practice parameter: 2010 update. J Allergy Clin Immunol 2010; 126(3):477–80.e1–42.
7. Ridolo E, Martignago I, Senna G, et al. Scombroid syndrome: it seems to be fish allergy but... it isn't. Curr Opin Allergy Clin Immunol 2016;16(5):516–21.
8. Nassiri M, Eckermann O, Babina M, et al. Serum levels of 9alpha,11beta-PGF2 and cysteinyl leukotrienes are useful biomarkers of anaphylaxis. J Allergy Clin Immunol 2016;137(1):312–4.
9. Fox S, Park MA. Penicillin skin testing in the evaluation and management of penicillin Allergy. Ann Allergy Asthma Immunol 2011;106(1):1–7.
10. Fox SJ, Park MA. Penicillin skin testing is a safe and effective tool for evaluating penicillin allergy in the pediatric population. J Allergy Clin Immunol Pract 2014; 2(4):439–44.
11. Carter MC, Desai A, Komarow HD, et al. A distinct biomolecular profile identifies monoclonal mast cell disorders in patients with idiopathic anaphylaxis. J Allergy Clin Immunol 2017. [Epub ahead of print].
12. Kristensen T, Vestergaard H, Bindslev-Jensen C, et al. Prospective evaluation of the diagnostic value of sensitive KIT D816V mutation analysis of blood in adults with suspected systemic mastocytosis. Allergy 2017. [Epub ahead of print].
13. Braganza SC, Acworth JP, McKinnon DR, et al. Paediatric emergency department anaphylaxis: different patterns from adults. Arch Dis Child 2006;91(2): 159–63.
14. Simons FE, Gu X, Silver NA, et al. EpiPen Jr versus EpiPen in young children weighing 15 to 30 kg at risk for anaphylaxis. J Allergy Clin Immunol 2002; 109(1):171–5.
15. Korenblat P, Lundie MJ, Dankner RE, et al. A retrospective study of epinephrine administration for anaphylaxis: how many doses are needed? Allergy Asthma Proc 1999;20(6):383–6.
16. Campbell RL, Li JT, Nicklas RA, et al. Members of the joint task F, practice parameter W. Emergency department diagnosis and treatment of anaphylaxis: a practice parameter. Ann Allergy Asthma Immunol 2014;113(6):599–608.
17. Muraro A, Roberts G, Worm M, et al. Anaphylaxis: guidelines from the European Academy of Allergy and Clinical Immunology. Allergy 2014;69(8):1026–45.

18. Simons FE, Ardusso LR, Bilo MB, et al. 2012 Update: World Allergy Organization guidelines for the assessment and management of anaphylaxis. Curr Opin Allergy Clin Immunol 2012;12(4):389–99.
19. Simons FE, Ardusso LR, Bilo MB, et al. World allergy organization guidelines for the assessment and management of anaphylaxis. World Allergy Organ J 2011; 4(2):13–37.
20. Fleming JT, Clark S, Camargo CA Jr, et al. Early treatment of food-induced anaphylaxis with epinephrine is associated with a lower risk of hospitalization. J Allergy Clin Immunol Pract 2015;3(1):57–62.
21. Pumphrey RS, Gowland MH. Further fatal allergic reactions to food in the United Kingdom, 1999-2006. J Allergy Clin Immunol 2007;119(4):1018–9.
22. Xu YS, Kastner M, Harada L, et al. Anaphylaxis-related deaths in Ontario: a retrospective review of cases from 1986 to 2011. Allergy Asthma Clin Immunol 2014; 10(1):38.
23. Goddet NS, Descatha A, Liberge O, et al. Paradoxical reaction to epinephrine induced by beta-blockers in an anaphylactic shock induced by penicillin. Eur J Emerg Med 2006;13(6):358–60.
24. Lee S, Hess EP, Nestler DM, et al. Antihypertensive medication use is associated with increased organ system involvement and hospitalization in emergency department patients with anaphylaxis. J Allergy Clin Immunol 2013;131(4): 1103–8.
25. Lee S, Bellolio MF, Hess EP, et al. Predictors of biphasic reactions in the emergency department for patients with anaphylaxis. J Allergy Clin Immunol Pract 2014;2(3):281–7.
26. Scranton SE, Gonzalez EG, Waibel KH. Incidence and characteristics of biphasic reactions after allergen immunotherapy. J Allergy Clin Immunol 2009;123(2): 493–8.
27. Jarvinen KM, Sicherer SH, Sampson HA, et al. Use of multiple doses of epinephrine in food-induced anaphylaxis in children. J Allergy Clin Immunol 2008;122(1): 133–8.
28. Joint Task Force on Practice Parameters, American Academy of Allergy, Asthma and Immunology, American College of Allergy, Asthma and Immunology, Joint Council of Allergy, Asthma and Immunology. Drug allergy: an updated practice parameter. Ann Allergy Asthma Immunol 2010;105(4):259–73.
29. Brozek JL, Bousquet J, Agache I, et al. Allergic rhinitis and its impact on asthma (ARIA) Guidelines - 2016 revision. J Allergy Clin Immunol 2017. [Epub ahead of print].
30. Cox L, Nelson H, Lockey R, et al. Allergen immunotherapy: a practice parameter third update. J Allergy Clin Immunol 2011;127(1 Suppl):S1–55.
31. Seidman MD, Gurgel RK, Lin SY, et al. Clinical practice guideline: allergic rhinitis. Otolaryngol Head Neck Surg 2015;152(1 Suppl):S1–43.
32. Cox L, Larenas-Linnemann D, Lockey RF, et al. Speaking the same language: the World Allergy Organization subcutaneous immunotherapy systemic reaction grading system. J Allergy Clin Immunol 2010;125(3):569–74, 574.e1–574.e7.
33. Bernstein DI, Wanner M, Borish L, et al, Immunotherapy Committee, American Academy of Allergy, Asthma and Immunology. Twelve-year survey of fatal reactions to allergen injections and skin testing: 1990-2001. J Allergy Clin Immunol 2004;113(6):1129–36.
34. Epstein TG, Liss GM, Murphy-Berendts K, et al. Risk factors for fatal and nonfatal reactions to subcutaneous immunotherapy: national surveillance study on

allergen immunotherapy (2008-2013). Ann Allergy Asthma Immunol 2016;116(4): 354–9.e2.

35. Ober AI, MacLean JA, Hannaway PJ. Life-threatening anaphylaxis to venom immunotherapy in a patient taking an angiotensin-converting enzyme inhibitor. J Allergy Clin Immunol 2003;112(5):1008–9.

36. Tunon-de-Lara JM, Villanueva P, Marcos M, et al. ACE inhibitors and anaphylactoid reactions during venom immunotherapy. Lancet 1992;340(8824):908.

37. Lee S, Stachler RJ, Ferguson BJ. Defining quality metrics and improving safety and outcome in allergy care. Int Forum Allergy Rhinol 2014;4(4):284–91.

38. Mattos JL, Ferguson BJ, Lee S. Impact of quality improvement measures on the delivery of allergy immunotherapy: a 2-year follow-up. Int Forum Allergy Rhinol 2015;5(6):513–6.

39. Mattos JL, Lee S. Safety considerations in providing allergen immunotherapy in the office. Curr Opin Otolaryngol Head Neck Surg 2016;24(3):226–30.

Future Horizons in Allergy

Michael J. Marino, MD, Amber U. Luong, MD, PhD*

KEYWORDS

- Allergic rhinitis • Aspirin-exacerbated respiratory disease • Allergen immunotherapy
- Immunoglobulin E

KEY POINTS

- Testing of local immunoglobulin E (IgE) in the nasal mucosa using mucosal brush biopsy may improve diagnostic accuracy.
- Urinary leukotriene E4 may be useful in identifying patients with aspirin sensitivity.
- Recombinant allergens and alternative approaches to allergen immunotherapy may offer disease-modifying treatment with improved safety and dosing compared with subcutaneous immunotherapy.

INTRODUCTION

There have been numerous advances in the diagnosis and management of atopy relevant to the allergy-treating otolaryngologist. These include emerging technologies, new devices, and refinement of existing methods, and in many ways reflect an overall trend in health care toward personalized medicine.[1] At the diagnostic level, these advances will help to identify specific allergic conditions in a clinically useful way, and even differentiate these from nonallergic diseases with shared symptomatology. Improved diagnostic precision is in turn fundamental to delivering targeted therapies.

Several developments in the diagnosis of allergy and related nonallergic conditions may aid the otolaryngologist in identifying and differentiating specific entities. Local immunoglobulin E (IgE) in the nasal mucosa can be useful in the diagnosis of allergic rhinitis, and mucosal brush biopsy may make this a practical test.[2–4] Urinary leukotriene E4 (LTE4) can identify aspirin sensitivity among patients with different respiratory diagnoses.[5–9] Lipidomics[10–12] and microRNA expression in extraceullar microvesicles[13,14] allow for the identification of extracellular allergic biomarkers, and may complement the traditional identification of intracellular proteins. Furthermore,

Disclosures: A. Luong received consulting fees from 480 Biomedical, Aerin Medical, ENTvantage, and Medtronic and the department received industry research funding from Intersect ENT and Allakos.

Department of Otorhinolaryngology–Head and Neck Surgery, McGovern Medical School at the University of Texas Health Science Center, 6431 Fannin Street, MSB 5.036, Houston, TX 77030, USA
* Corresponding author.
E-mail address: amber.u.luong@uth.tmc.edu

Otolaryngol Clin N Am 50 (2017) 1185–1193
http://dx.doi.org/10.1016/j.otc.2017.08.014
0030-6665/17/© 2017 Elsevier Inc. All rights reserved.

oto.theclinics.com

nasal provocation testing with optical rhinometry may help to differentiate allergic and nonallergic rhinitis.[15–17]

The management of allergy may be improved through the introduction of targeted therapeutics as well as the refinement of existing treatments. Intranasal steroids and antihistamines are part of the traditional management of allergic rhinitis, and the use of these drugs is supported by clinical guidelines.[18] New delivery systems and formulations may improve the efficacy of intranasal steroids and antihistamines by enhancing bioavailability.[19,20] Recombinant allergens offer the potential to be a targeted therapy with modifications for increased immunologic properties and decreased allergenic activity.[21–23] Meanwhile, alternative administration routes for allergen immunotherapy, such as epicutaneous,[24] intralymphatic,[25] and sublingual,[26] may allow for enhanced patient convenience, dose reduction, and improved safety. Monoclonal antibodies, such as omalizumab and dupilumab, may be useful in managing allergic rhinitis, and might be particularly useful in patients with comorbid conditions.[27,28] Finally, intranasal capsaicin may represent a treatment option for a subgroup of patients with nonallergic irritant rhinitis.[29–31] The various advances in allergy diagnosis and management are summarized in **Table 1**.

DIAGNOSIS
Local Immunoglobulin E and Mucosal Brush Biopsy

Allergen-specific IgE is defining of the pathophysiology of allergic disease, and is, therefore, used as a marker for these conditions. Typically, serum IgE levels have been used in clinical practice. Testing for IgE in the nasal mucosa may improve diagnostic accuracy when assessing for conditions such as allergic rhinitis.[4] Furthermore, there is a subgroup of patients with detectable allergen-specific IgE localized in the nasal mucosa, but who have negative skin prick testing and serum allergen-specific IgE.[32] Obtaining nasal mucosal tissue biopsy from patients for the diagnosis of allergic rhinitis is a significant barrier to the routine use of local IgE levels.[4]

Mucosal brush biopsy has been described as a technique for the collection of epithelial cells, monocytes, neutrophils, and eosinophils in the nasal mucosa as early as 1988.[33] In that study, Pipkorn and colleagues[33] indicated that mucosal brush biopsy might also be useful for biochemical analysis. More recently, Reisacher[3] demonstrated that antigen-specific IgE could be detected via nasal mucosal brush biopsy, including patients for whom skin prick testing was negative. Cells are collected from the mucosal surface of the inferior turbinates with a cytology brush and IgE is harvested from the lysed cells. Microarray analysis of nasal mucosal brush biopsy are more sensitive at detecting IgE levels than standard in vitro IgE assays, and may improve diagnostic accuracy.[2] A limitation of this technique, however, is the rate at which IgE is detectable in nonallergic patients has not been well-defined. Overall, testing the nasal mucosal for local IgE using a minimally invasive technique such as mucosal brush biopsy may improve the clinical diagnosis of allergic rhinitis, particularly among patients with negative skin prick testing and normal serum IgE levels.

Urinary Leukotriene E4

Several recent studies have described urinary LTE4 as potentially useful in the diagnosis of allergic disease,[5–8] particularly for identifying aspirin sensitivity.[5–7] In 2006, Micheletto and colleagues[9] demonstrated that urinary LTE4 excretion increased in aspirin intolerant-asthmatics who underwent nasal provocation testing with lysine aspirin. A systematic review and metaanalysis by Hagan and colleagues[5] examined publications pertaining to the use of urinary LTE4 as a diagnostic testing for aspirin

Table 1
Summary of advances in the diagnosis and management of allergy

Technology	Application	Clinical Benefits
Diagnosis		
Nasal mucosa IgE	Quantification of nasal mucosa local IgE using mucosal brush biopsy	Detection of antigen-specific IgE in patients with negative skin prick and serum testing
Urinary leukotriene E4	Detection of increased urinary leukotriene E4 in patients with aspirin sensitivity	Reliable, safe, and objective identification of patients with aspirin sensitivity
Lipidomics and extracellular vesicle microRNA	Detection of immunogenic nonprotein species	Diagnosis through the identification of immunologically active species that have not been routinely tested
Optical rhinometry	Detect changes in nasal blood flow to specific challenges	Objective diagnosis of nonallergic irritant rhinitis with intranasal capsaicin challenge
Management		
Intranasal delivery systems	Liposomal topical steroid and antihistamine formulations, and exhalational delivery systems	Improve the distribution and bioavailability of medications delivered to the nasal cavity
Recombinant allergens	Allergens generated from engineered DNA templates	Selection for improved immunologic activity and safety
Alternative administration of allergen immunotherapy	Epicutaneous immunotherapy, intralymphatic immunotherapy, and sublingual immunotherapy	Improve dosing regimens to enhance patient convenience and compliance
Monoclonal antibodies	Targeted blockade of immunogenic proteins	Disease-modifying treatment of allergic disease and comorbid disease, such as asthma, nasal polyposis, and atopic dermatitis
Intranasal capsaicin	Blockade of TRPV1-SP signaling	Inhibition of a potential mechanism for nonallergic irritant rhinitis

Abbreviation: TRPV1-SP, transient receptor potential cation subfamily V, receptor 1 – substance P.

sensitivity. When urinary LTE4 was quantified by a radioimmunoassay technique, the sensitivity and specificity for the diagnosis of aspirin intolerant asthma were 81% and 79%, respectively.[5] A simple and accurate test for aspirin sensitivity would allow for the identification of patients whose management would benefit from medication avoidance, aspirin desensitization, and multidisciplinary treatment of respiratory and sinonasal disease. Furthermore, urinary LTE4 testing may be safer and faster than the current gold standard diagnostic test of aspirin challenge.

Lipidomics and Extracellular Microvesicle microRNA

The biochemical diagnosis of allergy has traditionally been focused on the identification of intracellular or cell surface proteins. MicroRNA contained within extracellular microvesicles and lipids, however, may be involved in cellular immune responses.[10,13] To this extent, lipids and extracellular microRNA could be alternative biomarkers in the diagnosis of allergy. Lipidomics is the technique of profiling cellular lipids for identification purposes, and has potential application for the identification of allergenic lipid molecule species. Bashir and colleagues[10] profiled lipids in 22 common allergenic plant species using gas chromatography–mass spectrometry and identified 106 molecular lipid species, which were compiled into a database. This library in turn can serve in the identification of lipid antigens. Furthermore, that study demonstrated that these lipid molecules stimulated cytokine expression in dendritic cells and natural killer T cells, affirming the role of lipids in the immune response.[10] Asthma patients were also accurately identified by profiling eicosanoids in exhaled breath condensate[11] and lipid species in bronchoalveolar lavage fluid.[12] Analysis of exhaled breath condensate in asthmatics demonstrated increased 5-, 12-, and 15-hydroxysteicosateroic acid and prostaglandin D_2 and E_2 levels.[11] Similarly, bronchoalveolar lavage in asthmatics (not treated with corticosteroids) demonstrated increased prostaglandin, lysophosphatidylcholine, phosphatidylcholide, sphingomyelin, and triglyceride species compared with normal controls.[12] Exhaled breath condensate eicosanoid profiling was also able to discriminate aspirin intolerant patients with 92% accuracy.[12]

Extracellular vesicles, which are present in most bodily fluids, may contain RNA and even allow for the transfer of genetic material between cells.[13] This transfer of RNA, through extracellular vesicles in the nasal mucus, may contribute to the local immune response in allergic rhinitis, and therefore be a novel diagnostic target. In a study of patients with allergic rhinitis, extracellular vesicle microRNA sequences were compared with those in healthy controls. Certain sequences were found to be increased in allergic rhinitis patients, whereas other sequences were decreased.[13] Similar findings were also demonstrated in a mouse model of allergic rhinitis, and extracellular vesicle microRNA levels were found to modulate interleukin-10 expression.[14] Both extracellular vesicle microRNA and lipidomics may represent alternative approaches in the diagnosis of allergy, and are contrasted from the traditional biochemical identification of proteins.

Optical Rhinometry

Optical rhinometry offers a method for objectively measuring nasal patency by using optical spectroscopy to quantify visible and near-infrared light absorption in the tissue. The optical rhinometer is, therefore, able to measure the volume of blood within the nasal cavity, and in turn the degree of nasal congestion.[17] Optical rhinometry has been able to detect changes in nasal patency after nasal provocation testing with histamine, oxymetazoline, *Dermatophagiodes farinae*, and capsaicin challenges.[15–17] Nonallergic irritant rhinitis was accurately assessed using optical rhinometry with intranasal capsaicin challenge.[16] This may offer an objective diagnostic test for nonallergic irritant rhinitis, and aid in differentiating these patients from those with allergic rhinitis, despite overlapping symptoms.

MANAGEMENT
Intranasal Delivery Systems

Intranasal steroids and antihistamines have been central in the management of allergic rhinitis, and their use is outlined in clinical guidelines.[18] Alternative drug formulations for intranasal steroids and antihistamines have been developed using liposomal particles, with the purported advantage of improved bioavailability.[19,20] These types of formulations have been described for budesonide[19] and fexofenadine.[20] New delivery mechanisms are becoming available for traditional intranasal steroids. This includes exhalation delivery systems, which may have improved distribution of medication to the turbinates and osteomeatal complex.[34,35] New formulations and delivery systems offer the potential for increased efficacy for traditional drugs used in the management of allergic rhinitis.

Recombinant Allergens

Recombinant allergens offer the potential to increase immunologic activity, while decreasing the side effects of traditional immunotherapy. There are several advantages to recombinant allergens that are directed at certain deficiencies in the preparation and administration of natural allergen extracts. Recombinant allergens can be tailored precisely to the patient's sensitization profile and avoid contamination with unwanted allergens that can occur in the preparation of natural allergen extracts.[21] Unwanted allergens in natural extract preparations can lead to new cross-reactions. Dosing can also be closely controlled, because recombinant allergens are generated from a DNA template, allowing for exact quantities of the recombinant molecule.[21] This process also allows for modifications to enhance desired immunologic activity of the allergen, while suppressing unwanted allergenic activity. Overall, these features make recombinant allergens a more targeted therapy over traditional allergen extracts.

Recombinant allergen vaccines have been studied for the treatment of allergic rhinitis in randomized, controlled trials among patients sensitive to birch and grass.[22,23] Patients treated with a recombinant birch allergen vaccine demonstrated improved symptoms and decreased rescue medication use.[22] Increased specific IgG levels were also observed in the group treated with recombinant birch allergen, and there were not any unwanted cross-reactions.[22] In a comparison group treated with traditional birch allergen extract, 3 of 29 patients developed new IgE sensitivities.[22] In a study of recombinant grass allergen, patients in the treatment group also demonstrated improved symptom scores and increased allergen-specific IgG.[23] These studies indicate that recombinant allergens may be an efficacious alternative to traditional allergen extracts, and be targeted to specific allergy profiles.

Allergen Immunotherapy Administration Routes

Allergen immunotherapy has typically been delivered through a subcutaneous route. Alternative routes of administration have been studied and entered into clinical practice, including intralymphatic immunotherapy, epicutaneous immunotherapy (EIT), and sublingual immunotherapy (SLIT). These other routes have been developed to address disadvantages to subcutaneous immunotherapy (SCIT), primarily related to SCIT dosing schedules. Shorter administration routines or more convenient approaches would improve patient compliance and the number of patients that can consider allergen immunotherapy as a treatment option.

EIT has been suggested as an alternative administration route to shorten the treatment duration by targeting antigen-presenting cells in the skin.[31] A study by Senti and colleagues[24] found EIT to be an effective treatment for grass pollen–induced allergic rhinitis, with improvement in patient symptoms for the 2 seasons after administration. In this study, the patients only received 6 weekly patches for EIT delivery, substantially shorter treatment duration than SCIT. There were, however, local adverse events at the epicutaneous site, including pruritus, erythema, and eczema.[24] Intralymphatic immunotherapy has also been suggested as a route with decreased treatment duration, and was demonstrated to have improved patient-reported symptoms, decreased serum IgE, fewer adverse events, and better patient compliance than SCIT.[25]

SLIT has entered clinical practice as an alternative to SCIT for patients seeking a disease modifying treatment approach. In 2014, the US Food and Drug Administration approved 3 sublingual formulations for use in allergen immunotherapy.[26,31] These include Grastek for timothy grass, Ragwitek for short ragweed, and Oralair directed at 5 grass pollens.[31] Recently, Odactra was approved by the US Food and Drug Administration for use in house dust mite allergy. The approved SLIT formulations have been demonstrated to be safe and efficacious in large, randomized, controlled clinical trials.[36–38] SLIT offers patients the advantage of at-home dosing after initial observation in the office for adverse events. Up to 75% of patients experience a local oral or gastrointestinal reaction; however, systemic reactions are rare and thought to be as low as 0.06% of administered doses.[26] Preseasonal and coseasonal administration is preferred for SLIT because this regimen may have the same clinical effect as year-round dosing, while minimizing exposure to adverse events.[31]

Monoclonal Antibodies

Monoclonal antibodies may have a role in the management of allergic disease, particularly in patients with comorbid asthma. Omalizumab is a monoclonal antibody against IgE and is indicated in the United States for the treatment of moderate to severe asthma. In a pilot study of patients with severe asthma and comorbid allergic rhinitis, symptoms of nasal obstruction, rhinorrhea, sneezing, and itching were reduced.[27] Of the patients in that study, 73% were also able to discontinue the use of medications for the symptomatic treatment of allergic rhinitis.[27] Furthermore, omalizumab may have efficacy in desensitization for multiple food allergies, including children with peanut allergy.[28,39,40]

Dupilumab, a fully human monoclonal antibody directed at the α subunit of interleukin-4 receptor (IL-4Rα), has been investigated in the treatment of atopic dermatitis and asthma. IL-4Rα blockade inhibits the activity of IL-4 and IL-13, and has reduced IgE levels in mouse models.[28] Dupilumab has reduced exacerbations in patients with moderate to severe asthma, and improved symptoms in patients with moderate to severe atopic dermatitis.[28] Furthermore, IL-5–blocking antibodies, such as mepolizumab, reslizumab, and benralizumab, have been investigated in severe asthma, eosinophilic esophagitis, nasal polyposis, and Churg-Strauss syndrome.[28] Overall, monoclonal antibodies offer patients the potential for targeted and disease-modifying treatments for different allergic conditions in the head and neck.

Intranasal Capsaicin

Nonallergic irritant rhinitis can mimic allergic rhinitis symptomatically, and be a source of treatment frustration for patients without identifiable allergy and failing traditional therapies. Patients with nonallergic irritant rhinitis may have an increase in the expression of transient receptor potential cation subfamily V, receptor 1 (TRPV1).[30] Intranasal capsaicin seems to block the TRPV1-substance P (SP) signaling pathway in the nasal mucosa, and therefore may be a treatment for patients with nonallergic irritant rhinitis.[30] A recent Cochrane review[29] examined the usefulness of intranasal capsaicin in the treatment of nonallergic irritant rhinitis from the available published evidence. Intranasal capsaicin was found to be a treatment option, and that symptomatic benefits may last up to 36 weeks.[29] The current evidence, however, was based on several small, generally low-quality studies, and larger randomized controlled trials are needed to firmly establish the role of intranasal capsaicin in the treatment of nonallergic irritant rhinitis.[29]

SUMMARY

The otolaryngologist treating allergy can expect several advances in the diagnosis and management of this and related diseases. These advancements in both diagnosis and management will parallel broader trends in health care toward personalized medicine. Microarray analysis of nasal mucosal brush biopsies offers the potential to improve the diagnostic yield for allergy as the cause of rhinitis symptoms. In contrast, optical rhinometry may be a useful tool in differentiating patients with nonallergic irritant rhinitis. Urinary LTE4 levels can help to identify the subset of patients with aspirin sensitivity. Lipidomics and extracellular vesicle microRNA represent an entirely different approach to the diagnosis of allergic conditions, and uncover diagnostic gaps in the traditional identification of cellular proteins. Collectively, these advances would improve precision in the diagnosis of allergic diseases, the foundation for targeted therapies.

Management of allergy will be improved by the refinement of existing techniques, including improved delivery systems and formulations for intranasal medications. Furthermore, alternative routes of allergen immunotherapy may improve the efficacy, safety, and convenience of this option for patients selecting disease-modifying treatment. In keeping with trends for personalized medicine, multiple target therapies are becoming available to patients. These options include recombinant allergens selected to meet a patient's specific allergic profile, and developed for maximal immunogenicity. Monoclonal antibodies can also offer targeted therapies for a diverse array of allergic and related conditions including allergic rhinitis, food allergy, asthma, and atopic dermatitis. Last, intranasal capsaicin can be a specific treatment for patients with nonallergic irritant rhinitis, and allow for the successful management of these patients with related symptomatology.

There are multiple exciting developments in the treatment of allergy, and these promise to aid the otolaryngologist in treating these patients. Diagnostic techniques promise to bring improved precision, which in turn allows for directed therapies. To this extent otolaryngologists will be able to precisely diagnosis patients and offer treatments targeted for the specific allergic condition.

REFERENCES

1. Anaya JM, Duarte-Rey C, Sarmiento-Monroy JC, et al. Personalized medicine. Closing the gap between knowledge and clinical practice. Autoimmun Rev 2016;15:833–42.
2. Reisacher WR. Detecting local immunoglobulin E from mucosal brush biopsy of the inferior turbinates using microarray analysis. Int Forum Allergy Rhinol 2013; 3:399–403.
3. Reisacher WR. Mucosal brush biopsy testing of the inferior turbinate to detect local, antigen-specific immunoglobulin E. Int Forum Allergy Rhinol 2012;2:69–74.
4. De Schryver E, Devuyst L, Derycke L, et al. Local immunoglobulin e in the nasal mucosa: clinical implications. Allergy Asthma Immunol Res 2015;7:321–31.
5. Hagan JB, Laidlow TM, Divekar R, et al. Urinary leukotriene E4 to determine aspirin intolerance in asthma: a systematic review and meta-analysis. J Allergy Clin Immunol Pract 2017;5(4):990–7.e1.
6. Divekar R, Hagan J, Rank M, et al. Diagnostic utility of urinary LTE4 in asthma, allergic rhinitis, chronic rhinosinusitis, nasal polyps, and aspirin sensitivity. J Allergy Clin Immunol Pract 2016;4:665–70.
7. Yamaguchi T, Ishii T, Yamamoto K, et al. Differences in urinary leukotriene E4 levels and distribution of eosinophils between chronic rhinosinusitis patients with aspirin-intolerant and -tolerant asthma. Auris Nasus Larynx 2016;43:304–8.

8. Chiu CY, Tsai MH, Yao TC, et al. Urinary LTE4 levels as a diagnostic marker for IgE-mediated asthma in preschool children: a birth cohort study. PLoS One 2014;9:e115216.

9. Micheletto C, Tognella S, Visconti M, et al. Changes in urinary LTE4 and nasal functions following nasal provocation test with ASA in ASA-tolerant and -intolerant asthmatics. Respir Med 2006;100:2144–50.

10. Bashir MEH, Lui JH, Palnivelu R, et al. Pollen lipidomics: lipid profiling exposes a notable diversity in 22 allergenic pollen and potential biomarkers of the allergic immune response. PLoS One 2013;8:e57566.

11. Sanak M, Gielicz A, Bochenek G, et al. Targeted eicosanoid lipidomics of exhaled breath condensate provide a distinct pattern in the aspirin-intolerant asthma phenotype. J Allergy Clin Immunol 2011;127:1141–7.

12. Kang YP, Lee WJ, Hong JY, et al. Novel approach for analysis of bronchoalveolar lavage fluid (BALF) using HPLC-QTOF-MS-based lipidomics: lipid levels in asthmatics and corticosteroid-treated asthmatic patients. J Proteome Res 2014;13:3919–29.

13. Wu G, Yang G, Zhang R, et al. Altered microRNA expression profiles of extracellular vesicles in nasal mucus from patients with allergic rhinitis. Allergy Asthma Immunol Res 2015;7:449–57.

14. Luo X, Han M, Liu J, et al. Epithelial cell-derived micro RNA-146a generates interleukin-10-producing monocytes to inhibit nasal allergy. Sci Rep 2015;5:15937.

15. Luong A, Cheung EJ, Citardi MJ, et al. Evaluation of optical rhinometry for nasal provocation testing in allergic and nonallergic subjects. Otolaryngol Head Neck Surg 2010;143:284–9.

16. Lambert EM, Patel CB, Fakhri S, et al. Optical rhinometry in nonallergic irritant rhinitis: a capsaicin challenge study. Int Forum Allergy Rhinol 2013;3:795–800.

17. Cheung EJ, Citardi MJ, Fakhri S, et al. Comparison of optical rhinometry to acoustic rhinometry using nasal provocation testing with dermatophagoides farinae. Otolaryngol Head Neck Surg 2010;143:290–3.

18. Seidman MD, Gurgel RK, Lin SY, et al. Clinical practice guideline: allergic rhinitis. Otolaryngol Head Neck Surg 2015;152:S1–43.

19. Kim JE, Cho HJ, Kim DD. Budesonide/cyclodextrin complex-loaded lyophilized microparticles for intranasal applications. Drug Dev Ind Pharm 2014;40:743–8.

20. Qiang F, Shin HJ, Lee BJ, et al. Enhanced systemic exposure of fexofenadine via the intranasal administration of chitosan-coated liposome. Int J Pharm 2007;430:161–6.

21. Valenta R, Niederberger V. Recombinant allergens for immunotherapy. J Allergy Clin Immunol 2007;119:826–30.

22. Pauli G, Larsen TH, Horak F, et al. Efficacy of recombinant birch pollen vaccine for the treatment of birch-allergic rhinoconjunctivitis. J Allergy Clin Immunol 2009;122:951–60.

23. Jutel M, Jaeger L, Suck R, et al. Allergen-specific immunotherapy with recombinant grass pollen allergens. J Allergy Clin Immunol 2005;116:608–13.

24. Senti G, von Moos S, Tay F, et al. Epicutaneous allergen-specific immunotherapy ameliorates grass pollen–induced rhinoconjunctivitis: a double-blind, placebo-controlled dose escalation study. J Allergy Clin Immunol 2012;129:128–35.

25. Senti G, Prinz Vavricka BM, Erdmann I, et al. Intralymphatic allergen administration renders specific immunotherapy faster and safer: a randomized controlled trial. Proc Natl Acad Sci U S A 2008;105:17908–12.

26. Li JT, Bernstein DI, Calderon MA, et al. Sublingual grass and ragweed immunotherapy: clinical considerations—a PRACTALL consensus report. J Allergy Clin Immunol 2016;137:369–76.
27. Masieri S, Cavaliere C, Begvarfaj E, et al. Effects of omalizumab therapy on allergic rhinitis: a pilot study. Eur Rev Med Pharmacol Sci 2015;20:5249–55.
28. Ozdemir C. Monoclonal antibodies in allergy; updated applications and promising trials. Recent Pat Inflamm Allergy Drug Discov 2015;9:54–65.
29. Gevorgyan A, Segboer C, Gorissen R, et al. Capsaicin for non-allergic rhinitis. Cochrane Database Syst Rev 2015;(7):CD010591.
30. Van Gerven L, Alpizar YA, Wouters MM, et al. Capsaicin treatment reduces nasal hyperreactivity and transient receptor potential cation channel subfamily V, receptor 1 (TRPV1) overexpression in patients with idiopathic rhinitis. J Allergy Clin Immunol 2014;133:1332–9, 1339.e1–3.
31. Ricketti PA, Alandijani S, Lin CH, et al. Investigational new drugs for allergic rhinitis. Expert Opin Investig Drugs 2017;26:279–92.
32. Rondón C, Doña I, López S, et al. Seasonal idiopathic rhinitis with local inflammatory response and specific IgE in absence of systemic response. Allergy 2008; 63:1352–8.
33. Pipkorn U, Karlsson G, Enerbäck L. A brush method to harvest cells from the nasal mucosa for microscopic and biochemical analysis. J Immunol Methods 1988;112:37–42.
34. Palmer J, Jacobson K, Messina J, et al. Exhance-12: a one year study of safety and efficacy of opn-375, a fluticasone exhalation delivery system (FLU-EDS), in patients with chronic rhinosinusitis with and without polyps. Poster presented at: American Rhinologic Society Annual Meeting. San Diego (CA), September 16, 2016.
35. Optinose. Technical overview. Available at: http://www.optinose.com/optinose-platform/techcnical-overview. Accessed June 27, 2017.
36. Creticos PS, Esch RE, Couroux P, et al. Randomized, double-blind, placebo-controlled trial of standardized ragweed sublingual-liquid immunotherapy for allergic rhinoconjunctivitis. J Allergy Clin Immunol 2014;133:751–8.
37. Durham SR, Yang WH, Pederson MR, et al. Sublingual immunotherapy with once-daily grass allergen tablets: a randomized controlled trial in seasonal allergic rhinoconjunctivitis. J Allergy Clin Immunol 2006;117:802–9.
38. Didier A, Malling HJ, Worm M, et al. Optimal dose, efficacy, and safety of once-daily sublingual immunotherapy with a 5-grass pollen tablet for seasonal allergic rhinitis. J Allergy Clin Immunol 2007;120:1338–45.
39. Bégin P, Dominguez T, Wilson SP, et al. Phase 1 results of safety and tolerability in a rush oral immunotherapy protocol to multiple foods using omalizumab. Allergy Asthma Clin Immunol 2014;10:7.
40. Schneider LC, Rachid R, LeBovidge J, et al. A pilot study of omalizumab to facilitate rapid oral desensitization in high-risk peanut-allergic patients. J Allergy Clin Immunol 2013;132:1368–74.

Moving?

Make sure your subscription moves with you!

To notify us of your new address, find your **Clinics Account Number** (located on your mailing label above your name), and contact customer service at:

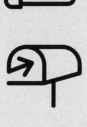

Email: journalscustomerservice-usa@elsevier.com

800-654-2452 (subscribers in the U.S. & Canada)
314-447-8871 (subscribers outside of the U.S. & Canada)

Fax number: 314-447-8029

Elsevier Health Sciences Division
Subscription Customer Service
3251 Riverport Lane
Maryland Heights, MO 63043

ELSEVIER

Printed and bound by CPI Group (UK) Ltd, Croydon, CR0 4YY

03/10/2024

01040394-0013